# Celebrating the Resilience of Queer Black Relationships

In a clinical landscape where traditional therapy models have historically been researched, constructed from, and designed for white heterosexual couples, this book offers an innovative framework to address the challenges, nuances, and strengths of diverse identities and relationships.

Drawing from Attachment Theory, Structural Family Therapy, Narrative Therapy, and the rich history and resiliency of Black LGBTQIA+ communities from the Harlem Renaissance to contemporary Ballroom culture, Multidynamic Relational Therapy (MRT) transforms centuries of wisdom and resilience into a practical five-step framework. This model specifically addresses issues of rigidity, power dynamics, and attunement in loving relationships while helping client systems break free from society's limiting scripts about love and connection. Through compelling clinical examples, Dr. Pennant demonstrates how this framework helps individuals navigate intimate relationships and generational trauma, moving beyond merely solving problems to achieve "Radical Emancipation"—the complete rewriting of relationship rules to create partnerships that are authentically their own.

This pioneering book provides clinicians with a versatile framework applicable to individuals, couples, families, and various relational constellations. It is an essential resource for therapists, counselors, and mental health professionals committed to culturally responsive practice and helping clients develop relationship patterns that honor their full humanity and unique relational needs.

**Anthony G. Pennant, PhD, CST**, is a licensed marriage and family therapist, systemic therapist, and is a certified sex therapist credentialed through the American Association of Sexuality of Educators, Counselors and Therapists. He is also an Approved Supervisor through the American Association for Marriage and Family Therapists. Dr. Pennant is an international speaker and skilled in working with neurodiversity, LGBTQ+ relationships, and foster care communities. As a passionate educator, his focus is on training couple and family therapists in the theory and practice of systemic intervention.

## Leading Conversations on Black Sexualities and Identities
Series editor: James C. Wadley

*Leading Conversations on Black Sexualities and Identities* aims to stimulate sensitive conversations and teachings surrounding Black sexuality. Written by academics and practitioners who have dedicated their work to the distinctive sexual and relational experiences of persons of African descent, the series aims to provoke an enhanced understanding throughout the field of sexology and identify educational and clinical strategies for change. Amplifying issues and voices often minimalized and marginalized, this series is a continuation and expansion of inquiry and advocacy upon the complexities and nuances of relational negotiation, identity affirmation, critical discourse, and liberated sexual expression.

Titles in the series:

**Sex Positivity and White-Sex Supremacy**
Ending Complicity in Black Body Erasure
*Carole Clements*

**Solutions For Anti-Black Misandry, Flat Blackness, and Black Male Death**
The Black Masculinist Turn
*T. Hasan Johnson*

**Black Women's Bodily Autonomy, Sexual Freedom, and Pleasure**
Explorations of the Hot Girl Movement
*Clarissa E. Francis*

**Butch Heterosexuality in Black Caribbean Womanhood**
Exploring Gender Performance and Sexuality
*Marsha Myrie Obi*

**Celebrating the Resilience of Queer Black Relationships**
A Guide to Multidynamic Relational Therapy
*Anthony G. Pennant*

# Celebrating the Resilience of Queer Black Relationships

## A Guide to Multidynamic Relational Therapy

**Anthony G. Pennant**

Routledge
Taylor & Francis Group
NEW YORK AND LONDON

First published 2026
by Routledge
605 Third Avenue, New York, NY 10158

and by Routledge
4 Park Square, Milton Park, Abingdon, Oxon, OX14 4RN

*Routledge is an imprint of the Taylor & Francis Group, an informa business*



ISBN: 978-1-032-72592-5 (hbk)
ISBN: 978-1-032-72597-0 (pbk)
ISBN: 978-1-032-72598-7 (ebk)

DOI: 10.4324/9781032725987

Typeset in Times New Roman
by codeMantra

Access the Support Material: www.routledge.com/9781032725925

# Contents

# Foreword

Dr. Anthony G. Pennant and I have known each other for a few years now as both of us belong to an organization that supports comprehensive sexuality education as well as offers credentialing for sexuality counseling and therapy. We met through a mutual colleague, and over the years, our relationship has grown in that it feels as if we are brothers. Our conversations have been rich, personable, and professional. It is not often that Black male professionals in mental and sexual health are able to meet and talk about leadership, influence, visioning, and systemic change. He is clinically insightful and strategic, and remains devoted to his clients and constituents. Conversations with Dr. Pennant are always easy in that he has graceful and inviting demeanor about him that allows people to feel comfortable sharing about a myriad of issues and experiences. Anthony is a once in a generation talent whose work has the capacity to influence not only Black and Brown therapists but also those who clinically serve these important populations.

Some time ago, Dr. Pennant and I talked about what may be the best medium for him to share his work with our community. We discussed the possibility of him authoring a book that captures some of his experiences as a Black male Queer therapist and the inherent professional and personal challenges that exist. There are not many spaces for this unique and profound perspective, and thus, I was happy when he agreed to contribute to the *Leading Conversations about Black Sexualities and Identities* series.

This book is written in a caring and authentic manner as Dr. Pennant provides us with case studies and vignettes that offer insight into working with diverse groups. This book embraces African philosophies, Person of the Therapist (POTT), and Multidynamic Relational Therapy that give practitioners clinical tools and options for supporting a variety of clients and their needs. Dr. Pennant's compassion is clearly evident in this book as he meticulously weaves his personal and clinical experiences throughout and offers us space to reflect upon how clinicians "show up" in and outside of therapeutic spaces.

This book can be used as an instructional guide to unpack and unravel the complexities and challenges of managing multiple intersecting identities and one's journey toward self-awareness.

James Wadley, PhD
Series Editor
*Leading Conversations about Black Sexualities and Identities*

# Acknowledgments

Being able to offer this body of knowledge to increase the safety and well-being of Black people, People of Color, Queer people, Queer People of Color, Black Queer people, and others in psychotherapy is a unique opportunity that I did not know would be given to me. I am filled with gratitude, excitement, and love. There have been others that have gone before me and many have given up their lives to sing the songs of liberation and emancipation that are visible in this book. I am thankful for the verses you weaved together. To the individuals and communities that led the way in us understanding the depths of expression and humanity in our sexual presentations, I am in awe of your wisdom. To Dr. James Wadley, I am extremely thankful for the ability to contribute to this series and for your guidance and support over the years. I look forward to seeing what amazing things you will do next. Much love to my professional friends and family throughout the United States and Europe keeping me grounded in what matters most and the string of memes, gifs (Annalise Keating GIF), and jokes that keep us sane and laughing. And last but certainly not least, my loving husband Courtney. You have always and continue to be a source of support and inspiration. You are one of the best things that have happened to me, and it has been a joy to embrace the fluidity and freedom of our Queer love. The future is wide open for us.

# 1 Intersectionality and Me

When I think about my need to write this chapter and all that comes with it, I feel extremely vulnerable. In my experience, most of my identities have been visible for all to see and do not have the option to be hidden. Likewise, some of my identities are hidden and others cannot see them unless I share them. Many of the said identities that are visible are ones that experience a great deal of oppression and prejudice and have been a pain point for me in my life. The most salient part of my identity would be my race. Even though I am multiracial, I am very much a Black facing individual. I am interacted with as a Brown person, spoken with as a Brown person, categorized as a Brown person and many times maligned as a Brown person. The color of my skin gives me such joy, but it is not always appreciated in the same manner as those I may interact with in the world. Being a Black person has been hard and is especially challenging as the history of the United States (where I currently reside at the writing of this book) and world seems hellbent on reminding folx that are not non-white that they are subhuman in some form or another. The passing of laws that seek to erase the history of genocide, native languages, family histories, and pain is rooted in white supremacy of which my skin color is the opposite of those that hold power. Race has been and will most likely always be an issue that is arduous for me to hold, handle, accept, and live with as the external factors are debilitating and impacting my very being.

In addition to race, another salient identity for me is my sexual orientation. I am gay and enjoy my attraction to other men and the male form in all its glory. Despite the advancement of LGBT+ rights in the United States in the last ten years where marriage equality was passed, and the repeal of Don't Ask, Don't Tell, and significant protections passed in various states for those who identify as LGBT+, the vitriol against my sexual orientation remains a visceral reminder that there are people who believe they have a right to hate who I am and many times will stop at nothing to exercise that right under the guise of their spiritual beliefs. The dominant narratives that I have endured regarding my gayness was and is to this day that my sexual orientation is wrong; needing to be rebuked and that it is impossible for two men to form a healthy relationship built on respect, love, affection, pleasure, and sexual satisfaction.

DOI: 10.4324/9781032725987-1

Lastly, I am a first-generation American. I straddle two worlds which overlap and complement each other on a good day but often are conflictual and battle for seniority especially during important decisions around values and the direction of interpersonal relationships and self-development. There are times when I am thankful for all the lessons and experiences that come from being a British Jamaican (among other ethnicities) descendant. Not only can I travel to the Caribbean as a citizen when I please, the richness of the culture and traditions around family and engagement with the world around you have informed my understanding and compassion for the world and community. In addition, the ability to not be bound by time or constraints of time shines through for me as the son of a Jamaica. I love to take my time and remove myself from the demands of production and instantaneous work where rules, emails, and tasks are ever piling up. There is a saying that in Jamaica, there are only two speeds, slow and stop and this perfectly describes how this culture greatly influenced me to appreciate how to live in the moment and truly be mindful about my relationship with time. It is my hope that Jamaican culture can catch up in affirming gay people as much as I affirm Jamaican life. Alternatively, I am also an American. I too have freedom of travel, and in many places of the world, my citizenship grants me immunity to many judgments even as a Black facing individual. In addition, as an American, I am the dream that many of my ancestors foretold. Many of them toiled and labored (some not by choice) to gain income and advance their children and give them the opportunity to thrive. I am the fruit of those labors. I have completed my PhD in Marriage and Family Therapy, teach in a graduate program, have become competent in treating and advocating for various issues and communities, and am writing this book.

Many times, I forget that I may have exceeded what my ancestors had envisioned for me as an American and for that I am extremely grateful. In contrast, these two citizenships often are conflicted and fight to be dominant. To operate in a space as a Jamaican does not vibe well as an American.

I describe some of the racial, cultural, and sexual orientations that I subscribe to as they are important to me and offer perspective for rationale and why this book was written. There is also one aspect of my identity that I think is important to share about where and who I am, and that has to do with my gender identity. I do have the privilege of being cisgendered and understand that there are individuals in our current society who do not and are not given the free pass to express their gender identity without oppression.

This is something that has assisted me in identifying ways in which I have privilege and where I have oppression. Being cisgendered in our society allows folks to exist in a place where their gender identity is not called into question. You need to know where I come from and who I am in this world, because my story shapes every word that follows. I have many areas of privilege, and I have many areas of oppression.

There is always a balance that must be struck between where and how I exist because my existence may be threatened at the drop of a hat. And many times, I have power to throw off those who would try to oppress me based on areas of privilege that I have. It is important to understand that when doing any work around intimate relationships and individual development and any kind of relational work, we understand ourselves. We understand how our self will clash into the other selves of those in which we serve and support.

The awareness that one must have around how they choose to support and/or intervene within people's problems and issues must always be tempered with an understanding that our things, our issues, and our beliefs perhaps won't influence too heavily the trajectory of wellness for those who we serve.

The work of a therapist is heavily aligned around some of the therapist's work. My journey of understanding who I was and who I am and perhaps who I am to become heavily aligns around the Person of the Therapist framework, but it also has been aligned from understanding my experiences of my identities, how my power has come about, and where I might make decisions that either supports how I move through the world or not. These journeys have created in part, the framework of the model of this book in which many Black Queer folx like me find ourselves in similar situations.

This model lives within my bones and I am confident that there are clients and therapists who have been waiting for a model like this that speaks their language. This is not to disparage the other models of couples' work and/or intimate relationships where heterosexual individuals are centered and research then supports that it is applicable in Queer communities. This is also not to disparage some of the work in which these models have enlightened us into the struggles of intimate relationships.

However, to have a model that is made and born from Queer Black identities helps our field concentrate on centering the most disenfranchised, oppressed individuals and to center their view of wellness, their view of health, and their view of connection. Putting this as a primary focus allows us as therapists to do two things to validate that life and that experience but also to show that they matter, that we matter, and that I matter.

The field of psychotherapy must move forward in being able to treat those who come into our offices, those who come into our screens, those who we supervise, and those who we see the entirety of them, to practice from a model that validates their existence and that uplifts them in all their capacities.

Long gone are the days in which we can no longer talk about race or power or gender or ethnicity and the impact that this has on our clients and intimate relationships and ourselves. Trying to do so gives problems much more of a space to fester and grow in our therapy rooms. I am laying myself completely out there, standing on business by putting my entirety on these pages because it needs to be reinforced that Queer love is healthy love. I hope that this book can prepare therapists to be trained more efficiently to help meet the needs of Queer and Black individuals and their relationships.

# 2 African Philosophy of Self and Person of the Therapist

We all have a pattern on how we keep our relationships and how we "show up" in relationships. These patterns and the relational ways we manage the interpersonal space between us and others are born from adversity, success, safety, and danger. These patterns are seared into our being and do not dissipate when we enter the therapy room as therapists. There is a prevailing and classical theory in the field of psychotherapy that describes the subconscious relationship between therapist and client: transference and countertransference. These phenomena were made popular by psychoanalysts like Freud (Prasko et al., 2022) who urged clinicians in their philosophy to understand that clients project onto their therapists as a part of the therapeutic process and therapist should limit their own projection of their own issues on the client. This philosophy is further elevated by other theorist that prescribe the way to manage the self in therapy as a therapist is to be a "blank slate." By emptying the self, the client's projection can be a mirror back to them which can support processing of deeper feelings (Arlow, 1995).

While these philosophies have been useful to the field, they are one-dimensional and limited and ignore philosophies from communities of color that expand on the self and the connections we have with our environment and other relational systems. One example of a differing philosophy of the self-rooted in communities of color are the concepts of Ubuntu. Succinctly, the definition of Ubuntu is "affirms that one becomes a human by recognizing the humanity of others…" (Mkabela, 2015). This key distinction on how we manifest ourselves as humans is entirely connected to our connection with others. We are deeply connected to each other and the ways we care for each other, speak with each other, serve each other, are served by others, share our feelings, and connect in our customs give us connection and meaning. Likewise, the Indigenous Wholistic Framework (Absolon, 2010) offers a similar understanding of the self. The individual is interconnected with various communities (home, family, tribe, country, education, etc.) with physical, emotional, intellectual, and spiritual information flowing in a multidirectional manner informing all who are connected.

DOI: 10.4324/9781032725987-2

These views of the self deepen our understanding of the interconnectedness and humanity of being a human being and are not readily appreciated nor centered as the norm in graduate-level training programs for counselors, therapists, psychologists, doctors, or psychiatric nurses. However, there does exist a framework regarding the self that seeks to incorporate many of the concepts of the self found with in Ubuntu and the Indigenous Wholistic Framework, the POTT model.

The POTT model is a framework made popular by Harry Aponte. Dr. Aponte found that clinicians needed more support in the "person practice" connecting the therapeutic interventions put in place for clients to the actual practitioner themselves (Aponte, 2016). Circa the year 2000, Dr. Aponte in conjunction with the Couple and Family Therapy program at Drexel University housed the beginnings of the POTT program where students in training could understand the important connection of the self and their practice of therapy. Two students who have undergone training in the model wrote a paper on their reflections of the training and highlighted their personal and professional growth in the program and in their practice (Aponte & Kissil, 2014). Moving forward from this chapter, the impact of POTT grew and more clinicians were trained under this framework.

The POTT model is a necessary addition to the practice of Multidynamic Relational Therapy (MRT) as it complements the application of the model creating authenticity of therapist interaction and intervention with the client system. All individuals in therapy appreciate genuine relationships with their therapists as this aids in the trust-building process, however, diverse, and vulnerable communities, such as the Queer community, require this to be in place due to external threat toward their bodies and well-being (homophobia, transphobia, misogyny, antisemitism, anti-blackness). The need for this has been amplified due to the rise in aggressive and oppressive ideologies that are rooted in white supremacy all over the world and recently within the United States.

The POTT model rests upon three pillars and the insightful understanding of the self. The totality of who we are, how we are, how we are connected, the decisions we make in relationships and how we respond to them, and many more actions lives within something called Signature Themes. These Signature Themes are relational patterns that appear for us in all relationships including the therapy room. Sometimes these patterns are born of hardships, sometimes they are born because of our personalities, or sometimes they are born from other factors. Signature Themes as therapists often become blind spots in therapy and cause us to over-care for clients and under-respond to clinical issues as we may be avoiding conflict with a relational pattern that hits too close to home for us or an area that we currently still struggle with. Much of this is congruent with the definition of countertransference; however, the understanding of Signature Themes and their subcomponent, wounded healers also have a useful function for the therapist. We as therapist can channel the energy we feel around these patterns for the betterment of our clients. The concept of a wounded healer helps us use ourselves and our personal experiences as powerful tools in how we share ourselves. Clients, intimate relationships, and families present vulnerable narratives and issues in their lives that are wounds that are slow and painful to heal. Pain and discomfort are both universal human experiences. A therapists own understanding of these issues and how they may impact life can be powerful tools linking clinical intervention, the self of the therapist and lived experience. In summation, the concept of therapists being wounded healers allows us to travel the road of therapeutic healing as companions on this journey through the use of themselves and not an uninvolved individual.

Building on top of the Signature Theme, the POTT framework has three pillars that guide the therapists understanding, development, and use of the model. Those pillars are the Knowledge of Self, the Access of Self, and the Use of Self. The synergistic and inter-reliance of these pillars provide the therapist the ability to reliably attune to the client system in front of them while managing themself in the real time. The ability to accomplish this provides therapists an opportunity to manage countertransference, pay attention to clinical issues present in therapy, and be accountable for issues of bias that can impact the therapeutic relationship.

There is a reason that most therapy programs begin students in Family of Origin or Personal History classes at the beginning of their plans of study. Being aware of yourself, who you are, your journey in life thus far, and even the issues that have been conquered are valuable data points that offer us an understanding of our lives. Knowing oneself provides an awareness of the issues that are present in our lives and gives us context to begin to understand ourselves. The journey of self-determination and destiny in all our lives comes into focus many times not when we know where we are going, but when we begin to take account for the things that make us who we are and how we respond to stimuli. This mirrors in part what happens with our client systems in the therapy room. They can learn more about themselves and come to accept who they are and what they are in control of (heightening a sense of agency). The Knowledge of Self gives the therapist a pathway to begin to understand who they are in the variable presentations of clinical issues and their relation to the type of therapist they are. This agency assists, in part, therapists with being flexible in how they view themselves.

The Access of Self is a real-time ability for therapists to ask themselves in the moment "What is coming up for me right now? How am I feeling at this moment? Is there something causing me to feel this way? I know I am feeling something(s) but I cannot figure out what it is." Being aware of oneself in the moment and building from the Knowledge of Self provides therapists the ability to many times manage themselves in times of anxiety, depression, distraction, excitement, and other emotions that bubble up and may interfere or compliment the intervention at hand. Asking these questions of ourselves and getting answers to them further the therapists' ability to be responsible for countertransference and clue them into areas that deserve more investigation with the client system.

The Use of Self is the final pillar of the POTT model and builds successfully off the growth and development of both the Knowledge of Self and the Access of Self. Therapists who are responsible for themselves can fully share themselves in the therapeutic process. We as therapist are valuable resources when delivering interventions to clients and a textbook delivery of the intervention itself falls short. Successful therapist and the treatment they deliver are flavored with who they are and understand it is not if you disclose in therapy but how you disclose in therapy. Lastly, the Use of Self allows us to actively turn toward our clients in need and attune to what they require in therapy. Does a client tell an instance of racism or sexism that bring up hesitation to respond in deep validation? Does a client share a story of abuse and isolation from their family that leaves them in despair and this hits home like you are telling the story? Does a client share the success of how they manage an emotional issue that is like your partner, your child, yourself, or a friend but you become muted as you do not know what is too much? These are all common experiences that arise in the therapeutic encounter that require us as change agents to respond in ways to lift our clients to the next level of their healing. While the MRT model heavily suggests that you become aware of this model and use it alongside its framework, POTT remains a powerful compliment to therapist training and practice.

The POTT model provides essential grounding for MRT's revolutionary practice. Where traditional therapy requires us to maintain distance from our clients, POTT invites us to bring our whole selves—our wounds, our wisdom, our liberation struggles—into the therapeutic encounter. MRT builds on this foundation by making explicit what POTT implies: our intersectional identities are not therapeutic dangers to manage but powerful tools for collective healing.

When I sit with Black Queer couples, my own journey with racism, homophobia, and family rejection is not countertransference to suppress—it is a source of empathy in action. MRT transforms POTT's self-awareness into active intervention. Knowledge of ourselves is just the beginning; we use ourselves as instruments of liberation. Every time we share our power, align our values, or choose joy despite oppression in our own lives, we become more capable of facilitating these transformations with clients.

This integration of self and system, personal and political, individual healing and collective liberation prepares us for MRT's radical proposition. Therapy that can heal wounds on the individual and relational level while also transforming communities and worlds. As we move into exploring MRT's five tenets, remember that this is embodied practice that begins with our own journey toward freedom.

## Exercises and Discussion Questions

1. How might your own cultural background and family of origin experiences influence your ability to authentically connect with clients from marginalized communities, particularly Black Queer individuals? What specific aspects of your "Signature Themes" might serve as both resources and potential blind spots?
2. Given the rise of oppressive ideologies, the text highlights the need for genuine relationships with therapists for diverse and vulnerable communities, such as the Queer community. How can a therapist use the POTT model to be accountable for their own biases and create a therapeutic relationship that is authentic and trustworthy for a diverse couple?
3. Discuss the interconnectedness of the three pillars of the POTT model—Knowledge of Self, Access of Self, and Use of Self—and explain how a deficiency in one pillar could negatively impact the effectiveness of a therapist treating a client system.
4. The POTT model emphasizes the therapist as a "wounded healer." How can you ethically navigate the balance between using your personal experiences as therapeutic tools while maintaining appropriate boundaries, especially when working with clients whose identities intersect with your own areas of healing?
5. Ubuntu philosophy suggests "one becomes human by recognizing the humanity of others." How does this contrast with traditional Western therapeutic approaches that emphasize therapist neutrality? What practical changes would you make to your therapeutic stance to embody this philosophy?
6. Consider a recent challenging session where you felt stuck or triggered. Using the Knowledge of Self, the Access of Self, and the Use of Self frameworks, how might you have navigated that moment differently to better serve your client?
7. How do you reconcile the individualistic training you may have received in graduate school with the interconnected, relational worldview presented in Ubuntu and Indigenous Wholistic frameworks? What systemic changes might be needed in therapy training programs?

# 3 Multidynamic Relational Therapy

Can someone tell me where the research on Queer people and their relationships is? Despite an increase in visibility of LGBTQ+ individuals, worldwide, the number of publications regarding Queer relationships remains elusive. Many of the major models of therapy claim that their model can be adapted to fit the needs of Queer folx and their lives (Healy, & Allen 2020; Westmacott, & Edmondstone 2020); however, there are no models of therapy that are built with the identity, dynamics, and relationships of Queer folx as the core of the model. As that is the current case, Multidynamic Relational Therapy (MRT) was created to fill this gap and provide a solid foundation for clinicians to be trained and attuned. MRT is a systemic therapeutic model specifically created to center Queer Black individuals and their relationships, operating through five core tenets: **Societal Expectations** (identifying and challenging harmful external pressures on relationships), **Values Alignment** (ensuring consensual agreement on core beliefs), **Power Analysis** (consciously sharing power rather than allowing domination), **Liberation** (actively challenging internalized oppression), and **Radical Emancipation** (fundamentally restructuring relationships free from oppressive constraints). Unlike traditional models that adapt heteronormative frameworks for diverse populations, MRT begins with the experiences of those facing multiple intersecting identities as its foundation, recognizing that Black Queer relationships have developed nuanced strategies for thriving despite systemic marginalization. The model emphasizes flexibility, allowing therapists to move fluidly between interventions as clients evolve, while aiming for "fourth-order change" that not only transforms individual relationships but extends into communities, ultimately empowering client systems to create authentic, equitable connections grounded in justice, mutual liberation, and the fundamental belief that LGBTQ+ relationships represent healthy, normal variations of human intimacy.

According to philosophical underpinnings of MRT, the presence of problems in one or more of these areas fuels discord and division in relationships and often limits solutions the people may have at their disposal to move past issues or overcome maladaptive relational dynamics. These problems do not stay in their own lanes. They spill over, mix, and concoct messier problems that you never see coming. For example, an intimate relationship consisting

DOI: 10.4324/9781032725987-3

of a cisgendered heterosexual couple who are white may find that they fight often around the roles of house that are tied to gender norms. A therapist may intervene and support first-order change around their behavior or even support second-order change by examining where emotional blocks on empathy and compassion lie within the execution of the roles. MRT goes further by specifically challenging how societal expectations on gender roles impact and influence people's ability to be free from said constraints and simultaneously enable third-order change by displaying these new revision roles (and the understanding) in the communities they reside in.

MRT is a model of therapy that was born from the dynamics of Black Queer individuals in intimate relationships. These relationships inherently face several oppressive forces against them due to factors such as race, ethnicity, culture, sexual identity, sexual orientation, and, sometimes, neurodiversity. The combination of some, many, or even just two of these identities in a heteronormative, neurotypical, and sexually rigid expectation in our communities creates hardships that often go unseen or even unimagined. This leaves people to be in states of high anxiety and hyper protection over their bodies and minds. An example of these interactions of identities colliding would be a Black Gay man. This individual is aware of racism and often is the subject of aggression (which may be verbal, physical, or both) toward himself from others simply because of his race. He may be profiled by the police, other authorities, or simply others based on the stereotypes of his skin tone. This person is also gay. While being a gay person has some support in the United States and in the world (Flores, 2019), there remains a significant number of places that would kill him on the spot based on his perceived or acted upon sexuality (i.e., kissing another man). When combining these identities together, a multitude of things may happen. In some LGBTQ+ places, he still may encounter racism and rejection from white LGBTQ folx. While he may journey to Black spaces, he may encounter homophobia and rejection from others in his community. This gay man also enjoys a level of privilege based on being cisgender and may not be threatened because of his gender express and alignment of his sex and gender presentation; however, this does not shield him from everything. Despite this, individuals similar in identity can find joy both in themselves and in their relationships and communities to which they are connected. Much of this is due to the flexibility of their roles and rules, the capacity to revision and reauthor their positions in the world, and the relationships they are connected to and the ability to identify and align their values. All these skills speak to their ability to survive, thrive, and flourish within relationships with themselves and others. The reality is that many of us navigate through many dynamics that impact our safety, well-being, and connection to our bodies and others — some having to navigate through much more than others.

A model of this alignment is, at least at the time of the writing of this book, is timely as the Queer community has made gains in being recognized within society (marriage equality and sexual orientation protection enshrined in law in many countries), and there continues to exist an active determination to both dehumanize and erase them. The recognition and utilization of this model by therapists is an act of advocacy and legitimization for Queer people. Increasingly, the individuals that mental health clinicians serve are diverse and traditional models of therapy do not center the identities of these individuals or contain interventions that promote autonomy and consent in their preference relational dynamic.

MRT embodies the next iteration of systemic psychotherapy and how the conceptualization of problems and the treatment of said problems are addressed in therapy. The model reflects a level of flexibility within the tenets that allow for a clinician to artfully move through and back again toward each intervention as the client system grows and changes. For example, a therapists may begin by examining and addressing Social Expectations that are causing negative impacts to the client system. From there, they may move into aligning Values as the Social Expectations of the system have shifted. With the alignment of Values addressed, the conversation on Power Sharing comes into focus. The addressing of power may cause the therapist to then revisit Social Expectations as the narratives of power may be connected to societal pressures. This in turn may cause Liberation to happen as the individuals are now free to redefine their relationship with a particular issue in a different way. This Liberation can then cascade into examining another Value or evaluate Power as the client system has changed for the better and seeks to level up. The therapist is free to fully embrace circular causality or recursive relationships (Kelledy & Lyons 2019) in the relationship(s) they are treating and the relationship the client system has with the therapist.

Fidelity to therapeutic models, specifically evidence-informed, and evidence-based therapies link their outcomes of treatment to therapists replicating the steps and orders of the model in the way they were written about and trained (Duppong Hurley et al., 2017; Ellis et al., 2010; Spengler et al., 2024). The reality is that therapists often change and/or modify their implementation of evidence-informed or evidence-based therapies in which they have been trained to meet the needs of the client system (Whiltsey-Stirman et al., 2015). There is also growing evidence that the battle between fidelity and flexibility in fidelity is a debate that is no longer important as data regarding client system outcomes generally are attributed not to the fidelity of the model but to factors such as therapist-client relationship, therapist belief in the model, and therapist training levels (Elliot et al., 2018; Fonagy & Luyten, 2019).

## Systemic Therapy

Systemic therapy, embodied by Couple/Marriage and Family Therapists (C/MFT) systemic therapists, can be described as a modality of therapy that focuses on individuals and their relationships. The systemic practitioner and their interventions focus on assessing, examining, and supporting the dynamics between two or more people to assist in addressing the issues that brought them into therapy. The philosophy behind systemic intervention existed well before the advent of Family Therapy in the 1950s and 1960s and could be found as a grounding and guiding relational ethos in many communities of the Global Majority—that is to say, the myriad of communities in the world that are collectivist in nature valued relationships between the self and others often prioritizing the group or community needs over the individual needs of one person.

The education and practitioner of systemic intervention are unique as they are adept in providing mental health treatment to an individual, any form of intimate relationships (couple, throuple, etc.,), and of course families. Special attention is paid to not just the content (what is said) but the context (the situational and external forces that impact folx) that shape relationships and their interactions. Questions and inquiries about the relationships of those they treat asked by systemic therapists are often circular in nature. They are the same questions asked to multiple members in the session often gathering more information about the view of the problem, how individuals feel about each other, the distance between them in relationship, the rules and roles of each person, and the dynamics that form interaction(s).

## MRT and Systemic Therapy

MRT is considered a systemic therapeutic framework as the theoretical underpinnings are focused not just on the individual but on the space between them. It seeks to move past the one-dimensional and behavioral-based interactions of cause and effect in behavior-based interventions as it is limited in outcome and does not incorporate the realities of oppression and relational dynamics that impact and shape our well-being. MRT seeks to elevate systemic intervention to incorporate aspects of justice and community change by ensuring that individuals become aware of their own personal dynamics and values and how those interact with others in their relationships and greater communities. Through this, a system of accountability and responsibility can grow within these networks and relationships by being attuned to both our needs and the needs of others, foster places to have difficult and challenging conversations, share power with one another, and build stronger relationships that are grounded health and wellness.

MRT also celebrates some of the most vulnerable identities in our societies and highlights the wonderful ways in which the Black Queer community have created a method to find joy, connection, love, purpose, identity, and community through their resilience despite the amount of oppression they face.

## What Are Queer Relationships? How Are They Different?

In the words of bell hooks, "Queer not as being about who you're having sex with (that can be a dimension of it); but Queer as being about the self that is at odds with everything around it and has to invent and create and find a place to speak and to thrive and to live" masterly sums up Queerness. Historically, Queer relationships have been described as relationships between same-sex individuals. This definition has widened over the years to include not just same-sex folx but other folx whose gender and sexual presentation are variable such as nonbinary, transgender, asexual, demisexual, and sides. Queer relationships and Queer sex often are expansive in function and rules as they have been seen as outside of what is "normal" in society. Queer relationships take pride, and rightfully so, in pushing back against the somewhat rigid dynamics of heteronormative cisgendered relationships which are organized around sex centering reproduction and not for pleasure; and roles in relationships being set by stereotypical categories of a person's sex and gender being the same. This is not to say that all heterosexual relationships align in this way; however, many of them align and often conform to these demands.

In Queer relationships, there is freedom to focus on what the folx within the relationship want or desire. Sometimes, this is focused on companionship that has meaningful connection on specific sexual roles, intellect, or division of labor (emotional, financial, etc.) more than on lines of gender. Other times, it is connection on sexual attitudes, satisfaction, and positioning where folx are free to engage with each other(s) to enjoy a variety of sexual positions, acts, roles, and other scenes which bring about sexual emotional satisfaction and connection.

Queer folx and their relationships have also represented a varied way of being and living that is seen not just as counterculture but also as a revolution against a thought pattern that individuals and relationships operate in a top-down dominating dynamic instead of one of equity, consent, and justice. Queer Black (and People of Color) relationships navigate the complexities of race, ethnicity, gender, and sexuality that often contain intricate and unseen challenges that both create hardships and increase creative ways for these folx to thrive.

## Theoretical Assumptions

As with all theories, assumptions tell us what the underlying reasoning on why systems operate in the way they do, why certain interventions cause change to occur within the we are supporting, how change occurs in the system, the common understanding of individuals being treated, and the ability for clinicians and researchers to engage in critical thinking within the boundaries of the model. For MRT, there are several assumptions which support clinicians on how to work within this model, its applications, and core beliefs about human relationships.

The first assumption is that clinicians have flexibility in applying many of the interventions of the model save for Radical Emancipation. While many theoretical models have deliberate steps laid out for the clinician to use in a linear fashion (and make room for some freedom), MRT seeks to free the interventionist to mimic the ways in which Black Queer individuals move about in their relationships; with freedom and flexibility to do things within an order that works for themselves and their interpersonal relationships. As stated previously, therapist flexibility and reflexivity in treatment intervention timing and even language used plays a critical role in successful attunement to client system needs.

Model fidelity in evidence-informed/evidence-based models provide clinicians for a roadmap on how to apply techniques and interventions for the client system; however, many individuals that present for therapy require recursive applications of interventions (Fonagy & Luyten, 2019) and flexibility in how therapeutic support is given. This point is magnified as interventions with neurodiverse humans who may require therapists and other helping professionals to tailor information in ways that are diverse and varied in both language and intent which may require interventions applied in a manner that makes sense for the client.

Like dancers who anticipate the beat to a song full of bass and life, therapists using MRT learn to move with their client system, shifting between interventions as naturally as the beat changes. While fidelity to therapeutic models does play a vital role in securing greater knowledge of a particular model, its relationship to better outcomes may not be as direct as professed within the world of psychotherapy (Fonagy & Luyten, 2019).

The second assumption is that this work centers some of the most vulnerable individuals within our society and global context, Queer people of color. The field of psychotherapy and psychological assessment and intervention are often norm behaviors and models in very heteronormative and white averages that then are checked for application with other populations. This model works in the other direction. Centering Queer Black individuals as the standard "average" supports moving the field forward in creating more equity and inclusion of models where clients can see themselves in the work being used by therapists. Notable persons such as Patricia Hill Collins, bell hooks, and Angela Davis state, through their lectures, writings, and lived experience, that if we as a society could work to support the most marginalized in our communities and build systems around them, then everything and everyone upward from them would be able to benefit also (Collins, 1990; Davis, 1971; Hooks, 2006). A model such as this can broadcast to Queer people of color that their identity and unique needs are not an add-on to an existing model but the central focus where they matter. This highlighted identity will also create a natural recruitment of folx of color and Queer individuals into the field of psychotherapy as they could practice within a framework that is identical to their lived experiences. Lastly, while this model is about Queer people of color, it can be used for all others and is inclusive of all other types of relationships and peoples.

The third assumption is that relational therapy such as work within intimate relationships and families requires therapists to have training in awareness of their own interpersonal understanding of themselves and the relationship patterns they keep. This is better summed up through the existing framework of Person of the Therapist developed by Harry Aponte (Aponte & Kissil, 2016). Therapists who can be knowledgeable about their family of origin, how they keep relationships, how they show up in the therapy "room," the access to their emotional state during sessions, and the use of themselves as a tool are far more prepared to attune with their clients. While all walks of life require a certain level of attunement by the therapist, Queer relationships require a higher level of this to ensure the space for therapy is validating to their experience and that the labor of understanding their walk of life is not on them to explain. Overall, the practice to have a greater understanding and awareness of a person's life and their own dynamics has a profound effect on their ability to practice and deliver effective therapy.

The fourth assumption is that this model is a paradigm shifting process for individuals and their relationships that help them transcend the barriers propped up in our communities that prevent people from exercising the power to control their lives, who they love, the roles they play, and the scripts they write with a great deal of creativity and flexibility. This paradigm is ushered in through the main intervention of MRT, Radical Emancipation. Therapists using this model should believe that the solution to some of the issues clients present with is often outside of the predetermined box of expectations or what we think should be the outcome.

The fifth assumption of MRT is that LGBTQ+ relationships are healthy relationships. The practitioner of this model must believe that Queer relationships are a normal variation of intimate human relationships, and that this variation is composed of and produces a flourishing connection(s). This assumption is vital as it mandates the relationship being seen as the center.

In the next few sections, we will visit each of five tenets through the treatment of a couple who presented for therapy. It is my hope that the explanation and application of this model is easily digested and understood by presenting it in this manner.

### *The Couple*

Lamar and Montana (pseudonyms) reached out to begin therapy as they desperately needed a therapist that understood issues in racial/interracial dynamics and sexuality. Lamar and Montana have been together for over five years and have been married for one year. Lamar identifies as a black cisgender heterosexual man and Montana identifies as a white cisgender heteroflexible woman. Lamar identifies as a black man and Montana as a white woman. Montana attends religious services regularly and Lamar does not. Their love story began in an accidental meeting that turned into a date that then morphed into a loving relationship. The two confirmed their intention for couple-ship and were soon engaged and wed a year later. The couple shared with me in our first few sessions their love story and the ways in which they demonstrated their adoration for each other. The couple also shared some of the tumultuous experiences that led to extreme difficulty in the relationship. There were three issues that stood out.

The history of microaggressions directed toward Lamar from Montana's family.

I A recent miscarriage
II Extreme fighting because of miscommunication
III Microaggressions toward Lamar from Montana's family

The goal(s) of the couple were to increase their communication, increase their capacity for empathy for each other, and connect better sexually. I affirmed these treatment goals and explained that I would be using the MRT model with them. Using MRT with Lamar and Montana revealed layers of complexity that traditional therapy models might have missed or treated as separate issues. While conventional therapeutic approaches might have addressed their communication problems through skills training, their sexual concerns through behavioral interventions, and the racial microaggressions as an external stressor to manage individually, MRT allowed us to see these presenting issues as interconnected manifestations of deeper systemic forces. The model's conceptualization of relational problems helped us understand that their "extreme fighting because of miscommunication" was more than poor communication skills. It was about how societal expectations around race, gender, and relationships had created invisible scripts that neither partner had consciously agreed to follow. Montana's struggle to support Lamar against her family's microaggressions was an issue about race, and it reflected unexamined values about family loyalty versus partnership solidarity that needed explicit negotiation.

### Exercises and Discussion Questions

1. The chapter argues that most therapy models claim adaptability to Queer relationships rather than being built from Queer experiences. Examine a therapeutic approach you frequently use—how might it inadvertently center heteronormative assumptions?
2. MRT emphasizes flexibility over fidelity to model steps. How do you balance evidence-based practice requirements with the need for therapeutic flexibility? What institutional or training barriers might prevent therapists from embracing this flexibility?
3. The model centers "the most vulnerable individuals" (Queer people of color) as the standard rather than an adaptation. How might this paradigm shift change your conceptualization of "normal" versus "diverse" populations in your practice?
4. The chapter suggests that centering Queer Black individuals benefits everyone "upward from them." How do you understand this concept, and what resistance might you encounter when proposing this approach to colleagues or supervisors?
5. How do the five theoretical assumptions of MRT challenge or support your current understanding of therapeutic change? Which assumption feels most difficult to integrate into your practice, and why?

# 4 Blackity Black with Some More Black in There

Being a Black person in this world is one of the sweetest and most painful experiences that a person could have. Black people in every part of the earth have had to deal with attitudes, laws, and sentiment that actively dehumanize them solely because of the color of their skin. They have been barred from entering places, having narratives assigned to them about their behavior or families, and have been subjected to being sold into slavery and have had their histories and lineage interrupted by being displaced, beaten, and broken. This legacy and narrative have had intergenerational impacts on Black communities that have come before the writing of this book and most certainly will continue after these words are read. The impact of these narratives around dehumanization is more than negative stories that are being removed from common conversations in schools and other educational spaces. They are being used to continue to "other" Black people, their bodies, and their initiatives and collective power and desire for equity and humanization in favor to further injure the said community. It is well researched that the Black community endures with ongoing racial stress (Hope et al., 2021; Jones, & Neblett, 2017; Jones et al., 2007) and other psychological impacts (Carter et al., 2017) that then left untreated and unvalidated are passed on to their children (Kaufman et al., 2023, p. 65).

There are many historical documents that highlight the past and ongoing issue around slavery and the populations that have been enslaved. These historical accounts speak on extensive systems in place used to supplement development and creation of their societies in exchange for removing their freedom. One such account is the transatlantic slave trade where approximately 12.5 million Africans were forcibly removed from their ancestral homelands, enslaved, and forced to procreate in the sole means of creating more enslaved beings (Black & Jackson, 2005; Stevenson, 2023). Many of the African slaves were subject to horrific conditions (being naked, not fed well, exposure to diseases, and packed in the boat like cargo) on the journey across the ocean from countries such as Angola, Nigeria, Sierra Leone, and Ghana. Once these slaves arrived at their destinations (anywhere to locations in the Americas and the Caribbean), these individuals were subject to further cruelty that ranged from maiming, whipping, lynching of family members

DOI: 10.4324/9781032725987-4

and friends, rape, family separation, and other cruel and unusual treatment (Douglas, 2011). Many of the 12.5 million Africans who were forcibly put in the transatlantic slave trade between the years of 1526 and 1867 (Black & Jackson, 2005; Stevenson, 2023) continued to have generations of children who were enslaved, had parents who were enslaved, and had children who were enslaved. The approximate 341 years contained times where original family histories and customs were lost, but others were created to maintain connection. It is not hard to imagine, but the intergenerational transmission of trauma (Carter & Barket-San, 2015; Comas-Díaz, 2016; DeGruy, 2005) was great and entirely rewrote experiences for these families causing damage to their bodies and minds. There were no official models of therapy to capture and support the impact of being bred and born in captivity and no framework around consent to help folx feel they had power to say yes or no to decisions on what to eat, having children, and where or who to worship and determine how they wanted to move through life. The anxiety, depression, isolation, and other unimaginable feelings around the catastrophe of being an enslaved individual and bringing children into the world that would also be enslaved is quite immeasurable and inescapable. There was no time to grieve when a loved one or community member died as you were seen as property and subhuman. The customs of life, death, community, faith, and the histories of wisdom and respect for the land forcibly replaced with versions of these human aspects that were more digestible, Eurocentric, and easily monitored. There is much more to describe of this ordeal yet; many of these Black people survived and found ways to dare I say thrive.

Much like the English Ivy, former slaves from much of the Ivory Coast and other places on the African continent found a way to root themselves and grow. People once known as being hailed from a specific tribe such as the Igbo were told they were Black or colored during slavery which denoted an opposition to being White. The contrast between being a Black person or a White person were characterized with being dirty, subhuman, unworthy, and unworldly (Black people) and clean, worthy, upright, and humane (White people) (Carter & Barket-San, 2015). Clearly these descriptors are untrue yet it was prevalent in thought that to be Black was less than in the human experience and justified to be treated as an other. The Black community attempted to redefine (Tate, 1998) in part the label of being Black to African American (which is still popular today); however, the more dominant identity and reclamation of being Black still reigns as a global identity.

The reclamation of the word Black and the power of being Black were in part made popular by the Black Panther movement. To be Black was something to be proud of. One could not change your skin color, but why would you want to? The skin we were born with provides natural sun protection. The color of our skin ranges from caramel to dark chocolate and provides such a striking contrast to many colors. Our hair comes in so many curl patterns that create opportunities for us to design our hair in creative patterns and styles. Our community often sets the tone on fashion, language, appeal, cuisine, and music. There is a sense of pride and honor when who you are, and the creative outlook of the expression of your being is a cornerstone of cultural symbols and identity across various communities. There is a sense of pride and acknowledgment when you can change the lexicon of engagement between people. There is hope for the future when your poetry, your concepts, and your declarations of humanity can articulate a way forward for the Black experience and dollar to be respected and valued as the same.

The Black Power philosophy lived differently within two main different social movements. The Civil Rights movement sought to create dialog between the Black and White communities and the US government (one could argue that this was the seat of power of White supremacy) to create legislation that allowed for full integration of Black people into the country with equal rights and access to services and space (Branch, 1988). The Civil Rights leaders did not necessarily agree with some of the methods used/preferred (some argued for more aggressive tactics); however, they all sought to demonstrate Black Power and mobility to advocate for inclusion into society and challenge the current power structure that thrived off of the suppression of Black folk in more peaceable and action-led terms (voter registration, boycotts, marches, and other grassroots community-organized demonstrations) (Hall, 2005).

The Black Panther Party, and other similarly aligned groups, sought inclusion of Black people into the larger community, but they departed from the Civil Rights leaders thought about peaceable and nonviolent incremental change (Jeffries, 2018; Newton, 1973; Van Deburg, 1997). The Black Panther Party and its parallel groups favored more immediate, aggressive, and impactful ways to tackle institutional racism and the structures that kept that power in place. Black Power was conceptualized as a pride in one's Black identity, skin color, and intellectualism that lead to encouragement in the creation of dedicated Black spaces. These Black spaces were beacons for Black people to exist in environments that nurtured a healthy relationship of themselves to their skin color. These Black spaces that contained Black Power taught and reminded them of their ability to have governing control over the bodies and communities. They also created dedicated educational arenas through cooperation with Historical Black Colleges and Universities (HBCUs) that proliferated Black Power through intellectual discourse, writing, and research (Joseph, 2006; Ransby, 2003). In addition, these Black spaces supported an ideological underpinning that Black bodies deserved the ability practice self-determination according to their own choices and highlighted that despite the historical atrocity against the global Black community, the autonomy and power over their lives still rested with them.

The Multidynamic Relational Therapy (MRT) model honors the Black Power movement and ideas about humanity via the philosophy of Blackness and borrows from its historical position on the narrative about the freedom to define relationships in the manner a person chooses. Throughout future chapters, the reader will uncover how and why Black Queer individuals and their relationships have and continue to be a template for healthy lasting relationships for all people. The language within the Black Power movement and Blackness give relational systems a framework to understand the power of self-determination for both the individual and the communities in which they reside.

The philosophy of Blackness and the legacy of Black Power movements do more than inform MRT; they are its lifeblood. When we speak of Societal Expectations in the therapy room, we channel the same recognition that led Black communities to reject beauty standards set by Eurocentric appearances and embrace the coil and bounce of Black natural hair as a crown on one's head.

MRT's Power Analysis draws directly from the Black liberation movement and their understanding that power that is hoarded becomes poison, while power that is shared can become a tonic to those in need. The Liberation tenet channels every ancestor who chose joy in the face of genocide, who danced despite shackles, and who dared to love despite whatever laws were passed. And Radical Emancipation? This is the therapeutic equivalent of establishing a Black Wall Street, creating HBCUs, and building ballroom houses—constructing new worlds when the present one denies your ability to exist.

When folx enter our therapy rooms, the goal is to not just treat symptoms or resolve trauma. We are opting into the long tradition within Black communities, making a way out of no way. Every Black Queer couple who learns to love freely despite society's restraints adds another verse to freedom for us all. MRT does not appropriate Black liberation. It transports innovative principles of justice into therapeutic practice, making the personal political and the political personal.

### Exercises and Discussion Questions

1. Given the intergenerational transmission of trauma from slavery and ongoing racism, how do you assess for and address historical trauma in your Black clients without pathologizing their experiences or reducing their resilience to mere survival responses?
2. This chapter discusses the reclamation of "Blackness" as a source of power and pride. How can non-Black therapists authentically support this reclamation process without appropriating or minimizing the significance of Black identity?
3. How do the different philosophies of the Civil Rights movement versus the Black Panther movement inform your understanding of various approaches your Black clients might take toward resistance and healing? How do you support clients who may align with more radical approaches to change?
4. Consider how the Black Power movement's emphasis on self-determination applies to your therapeutic practice. In what ways might traditional therapy models inadvertently undermine client autonomy, and how can MRT principles restore it?

# 5 Societal Expectations

No matter what way it is sliced, society has an influence on us. Many times, this influence is welcome and helpful as it creates a sense of belonging and acceptance and provides a common language to exemplify our experiences. For example, certain memes made from a housewife (receipts! proof! timeline! screenshots!) provide joy to folx as that scene provides a common language on what might be funny and how people are relating to pop culture. On the other hand, societal expectations can be limiting and oppressive, and many times, what may be an expectation or experience that brings people together may also cause harm.

Expectations are all around us. They are contracts and that we abide by and govern how we make decisions in part and shape our relationships. For some expectations, we opt into and understand fully what we are giving, what we are getting, why the exchange exists, and how to alter it if necessary. For other expectations, we do not consent to, they are hoisted on to us, and we are demanded to uphold the contract. Other times, we behold these expectations without consent and choose not to adhere to them. In all our communities, there are expectations that govern the dynamics of our relationships and impact our sense of belonging and connectedness. The expectations within the larger macro-communities such as the neighborhoods we live in, our places of worship, our cities, our states, and our country are powerful and have considerable influence. Many expectations are helpful and help provide consistency for us as we navigate life. There are several expectations that show up for folx and in society they operate as roadmaps

While the opinion of various relationships, interracial relationships (Campbell & Herman, 2015), Queer relationships, polyamory, blended families, multigenerational families, and single families, have differing levels of support, Black Queer relationships have been on the outskirts of what intimate relationships are to look like.

Our relationships and walk through this world are filled with intersections of societal expectations. It begins earlier than our birth hour. Our parents may be celebrating our sex, selecting our names, choosing our clothes, and figuring out our schools. We organize our social roles based around perceived and

DOI: 10.4324/9781032725987-5

enforced gender identity. We are told what family is, the conditions on how to connect, and the notion of giving our all, endlessly as parents. While many of these things are normal and encompassing our care, they can be predetermined and many times limiting to how we live our lives. Individuals turned couples and intimate relationships of all constellations into commitment with helpful and unhelpful societal expectations that intersect their relationships, dynamics, and life cycle decisions. Individuals in these relationships often have some conversation with each other about what their expectations might be in a relationship; however, the background of these expectations are often silent until a conflict occurs.

Black Queer relationships, like many others, have had social expectations about their relationships including the threat of being nonexistent, leveled at them for several years, yet they have found a way to rebuff these narratives. Multidynamic Relational Therapy (MRT) seeks to do this same thing, challenge unhelpful and oppressive narratives that masquerade as expectations, and allow intimate relationships to define the expectations they see fit for their relationships.

One of the preliminary and ongoing interventions and questioning with Lamar and Montana was the curiosity of the societal expectations they internalized that appeared to be some of the cause of their conflict. A specific example of this can be seen below:

*THERAPIST:* So, tell me, when you all fight about your fights, what is coming up for you all?

*LAMAR:* I am frustrated.

*THERAPIST:* Can you tell me more?

*LAMAR:* I feel like we do not communicate well and there is so much misunderstanding.

*THERAPIST:* Thank you for that Lamar. Montana, what about you?

*MONTANA:* I agree with Lamar, frustrated is a good word but I would add that I feel isolated. I do not know what he needs and he often does not give me room to find out how he may be feeling and how to fix it. I am his wife.

*THERAPIST:* This appears to be very frustrating for you both. May I use that word to describe how you are feeling?

*MONTANA AND LAMAR* Yes

*THERAPIST:* I wonder if there are two layers of issues going on that are causing this miscommunication. The first is the issue of permission and consent; the second is duty.

*MONTANA:* I am not sure what you mean by duty.

*THERAPIST:* Well, first, for both of you, when you are frustrated or feel like you are missing each other via communication, do you all share how you feel? Are you able to articulate what it is that you might want from your partner? The second is where does this urge to "fix it" come from?

*LAMAR AND MONTANA:* No (in unison).

*LAMAR:* I am too annoyed in the moment to even share my feelings most of the time and I certainly do not let her know what I want from her.

*MONTANA:* (Interrupting) Yeah, but don't you see that as the problem? Lamar, I do not know how you feel and I cannot fix any of it.

*THERAPIST:* (To Montana) Why do you need to fix it?

*MONTANA:* You do not understand. In my family, I was always held responsible to keep the peace and hold people's feelings. Things were chaotic.

*THERAPIST:* That sounds incredibly challenging and I can only imagine the impact on you.

*MONTANA:* It was hard being the only girl in the house. I was told that it is a woman's place to cook, to clean, to make everyone feel well, and to cheer them up. I hated that then and I hate it now.

*THERAPIST:* Why do you keep to that expectation? Is that something that Lamar asks you to or that you feel you need to continue to do?

*LAMAR:* I do not need her to do it.

*MONTANA:* No, I do not but I have never thought about leaving that behind…

Clearly, we see here that Montana endorsed a script from childhood that women should carry the emotional labor of those around them, specifically from the men in relationship with them. Challenging the societal expectation around women being responsible for the well-being of a relationship and the need to "fix" anything within the home was one of the major interventions with this couple. It allowed Montana the opportunity to evaluate not only the consent process of sharing her feelings but also the ability to change the "mandate" of how her perceived gender socialized her to exercise a duty to serve. When the therapist can support a couple to shift the basic ground rules of interactions that are based in presumptions that are not productive or hamper solutions, they are able to create additional manners to move forward in addressing issues.

## Societal Expectations—Clinical Application Exercises

### *Implementing Societal Expectations in Your Practice*

*Presession Preparation*

Before exploring societal expectations with clients, examine your own. What expectations about relationships, family, sexuality, and gender do you carry? Which serve your clients, and which might constrain them? MRT requires us to manage our own assumptions and lived experiences.

*Assessment Phase with Client(s)*

Begin with the Expectations Mapping Exercise:

1 Create three columns: "Expectations I Chose," "Expectations Imposed on Me," and "Expectations I am Unsure About."
2 Have each person fill these out independently (if working with a client system).
3 Compare and/or discuss answers, noting patterns, and surprises.

*Key Clinical Questions*

- "When you think about how relationships 'should' work, whose voice(s) do you hear?"
- "What would happen if those expectations went unfulfilled?"
- "Which expectations feel like mandates and which feel like foundations you can grow on?"
- "If you could refuse just one expectation, which would you rebuff and what you do you think the effect of doing so would be?"

*Intervention Techniques*

**The Expectation Assessment** (Figure A): Therapists are adept in exploring deeper connections clients have with presenting issues. Through the Expectation Assessment, we can excavate what may be below the layers of expectations:

- Surface level: Current relationship rules
- Historical level: Family of origin messages
- Cultural level: Community norms
- Societal level: Systemic messages

| ***Layer*** | ***Expectation*** | ***Source*** | ***Age First Heard*** | ***Cost to Relationship*** | ***Keep/ Release/ Modify*** |
|---|---|---|---|---|---|
| Surface | "We should have sex 2×/ week" | Magazine article | 25 | Pressure, performance | Release |
| Family | "Men don't cry" | Father | 5 | Emotional disconnection | Release |
| Cultural | "Keep relationship problems private" | Community norm | Childhood | Isolation, no support | Modify |
| Societal | "Gay relationships don't last" | Media/society | Teen | Fear, over compensation | Release |

*Figure A* Expectation Assessment

***Script: Challenging Inherited Expectations***

*For an Intimate Relationship/Family*

"I notice I am holding an expectation that [specific expectation]. When I examine its roots, I realize this came from [source], not from us. This expectation costs us [specific impact]. I want to explore what *we* believe about [identified topic] based on our values and desires, not inherited scripts. Do you find that this is the same for you? Are there other expectations you would like to identify?"

*For an Individual*

"I notice I am holding an expectation that [specific expectation]. When I examine its roots, I realize this came from [source]. This expectation costs me [specific impact]. I want to explore what *I* believe about [identified topic] based on my values and desires, not inherited scripts. I want to create expectations that I consent to and are healthy for me."

*The Contract Renegotiation*

Clients may appreciate substantive ways to verbally or by other means, declare that they wish to renegotiate expectations in their lives. A therapist may begin the conversation by reminding them as follows: "You've been living by contracts you never signed. Today, we write ones with your full consent."

Create actual contracts where folx explicitly agree to their chosen expectations and formally reject imposed ones. Not every intervention or expression of emotions/stances in therapy should be verbally based. Below are different methods to complete a contract renegotiation.

*Visual and Artistic Expressions*

1 **Contract Burning Ceremony**: Create visual representations of unwanted expectations by creating collages, drawings, or written words on paper. Clients can safely burn these "old contracts" while creating new, colorful artwork representing their chosen expectations and agreements.
2 **Sculpture of Liberation**: Using clay or materials such as Legos, clients build sculptures representing constraining expectations, then physically break them apart and reshape the remnants into forms that represent their authentic choices.
3 **Expectation Mapping Canvas**: Partners create large collaborative paintings with two distinct sections: one side shows imposed expectations in dark, heavy colors and restrictive shapes; the other side shows their chosen agreements in vibrant colors and flowing forms. A bridge or transformation area connects both sides.
4 **Photo Narrative Series**: Clients take photographs that tell the story of moving from imposed expectations to chosen ones—staging scenes that represent old constraints versus new freedoms, creating a visual journey of their relationship evolution.

*Movement and Dance*

1 **Expectation Release Dance**: Begin with rigid, mechanical movements representing imposed expectations, then gradually transition into free-flowing, authentic movement that represents the couple's true desires and agreements.
2 **Weighted Movement Exercise**: Use actual weights or resistance bands to represent heavy expectations while moving, then remove them and experience the freedom of movement, symbolizing the release from unwanted obligations.

*Musical and Sound*

1 **Vocal Ritual**: Begin by playing (and singing along should they desire) a song(s) that represent(s) the constraints of expectations that were thrust on them. Afterward, a song that symbolizes the freedom of their choices is played (again signing along if they are open to it).
2 **Rhythm Renegotiation**: Use drums or percussion instruments to beat out the demanding rhythms of imposed expectations, then create new, personally meaningful rhythms and beats that represent their chosen pace.

*Textile and Craft Arts*

1 **Unraveling and Reweaving**: Take apart existing textile pieces (representing old contracts) and weave the threads into new patterns and designs that reflect their conscious agreements and chosen relationship structure.

*Nature and Outdoor Expressions*

2 **Stone Release Ritual**: Find and hold stones while identifying old expectations the client wishes to release. To symbolically release them, either skip or throw them into water or bury them allowing them to rest. Clients can find other rocks and then pour their renewed expectations into them and decide if they want to keep them.
3 **Garden Replanting Ceremony**: Remove plants that represent unwanted expectations from a garden space, then plant new ones that symbolize their chosen expectations.

*Technology and Digital Arts*

1 **Digital Story Creation** Use video editing tools to create a short film showing the transformation from imposed expectations to chosen ones, using symbolism, metaphor, and visual storytelling rather than words.

*Common Clinical Challenges*

**Challenge**: "But our culture/religion/family says..."
**MRT Response**: "I honor that these beliefs have meaning. Can we explore whether they nurture or diminish who you are becoming together? Not all traditions should carry loyalty. There may be other ways that we can honor traditions in our families while also creating conditions to acknowledge them in modified ways."
**Challenge**: "We can't just ignore society's expectations."
**MRT Response**: "You are correct, we can't ignore them. But we can choose how much power they have in your private spaces. What if your relationship became an asylum from society's demands?"

*Session Flow Example*

Opening (10 minutes):

- Check-in about expectations they noticed during the week.
- Body scan: Where do expectations live somatically?

Exploration (25 minutes):

- Deep dive into one specific expectation.
- Trace its origins and current impact.
- Evaluate consent and utility.

Intervention (15 minutes):

- Practice rejecting the expectation.
- Role-play responses to external pressure to adhere.
- Develop boundary statements.

Integration (10 minutes):

- Create homework: Notice and document three imposed expectations.
- Practice one refusal.
- Journal about the feelings that arise.

*Documentation Suggestions*

Track which expectations are identified, challenged, released, and/or rejected. Note: Document somatic responses to discussing expectations as bodies often know that demands may be creating psychological distress before a mind can recognize.

## Exercises and Discussion Questions

1 This chapter distinguishes between expectations we "opt into" versus those "hoisted onto us." Think about your own experiences and list out expectations that you have opted into and those what were hoisted onto you. How did you personally reconcile with the expectations you have consented to and those you have not?

2 How do you address situations where one partner's liberation from oppressive societal expectations threatens the other partner's sense of security or identity? What does consent look like in the process of challenging expectations?

3 Black Queer relationships are described as existing "on the outskirts" of acceptable relationship models. How can you help clients transform this marginalization into a source of creative relationship-building rather than shame or isolation?

4 Consider your own societal expectations about therapy, healing, and professional relationships. Which of these might limit your ability to fully embrace the flexibility and authenticity that MRT requires?

# 6 Values

The word "values" could be defined as a set of beliefs or rules that govern how a person behaves. These beliefs influence how people make decisions and elevate what might be important. Values have an incredibly important role in intimate relationships, and shockingly, many couples do not speak about their values prior to their relationship commencing or know how to navigate differing values.

Values show up for us in a variety of ways and help us center what might be important in our lives. Within Black Queer relationships, values are discussed and managed consistently. From the declaration of sexual positions to the desire and decision on what family expansion looks like (to have children, expand intimate relationships, bring in chosen family) or how they privilege voice and history. The ability to discuss and manage the values comes from their lived experiences. Many times, Black Queer people have had to prioritize decisions that elevate their safety, preserve their history, or bring joy and happiness in the face of oppression and hatred for who they are. Existing in such a dynamic, while under distress many times, can impart a skill for rapid redevelopment and attunement to examine the things that are of importance and promote a need for cooperation to limit the amount of distress that one may experience.

Montana and Lamar had their fair share of values conversation in therapy sessions. As the therapist using this model, I had the opportunity to explore how their values intersected their relationship in various ways including values that they held and were aligned with, values that they held and were not aligned with, values that existed and they did enact or engagement with, and values that did not exist in their relationship and wanted to align and integrate. An excerpt from the session where values were discussed is below.

*THERAPIST:* So, today, could we talk through a few things? I would like to see where you all align on a few topics and I believe it could be helpful to our conversations and treatment.

*LAMAR AND MONTANA:* Sure.

DOI: 10.4324/9781032725987-6

*THERAPIST:* Have you all ever had the chance to speak about the ideas or beliefs on topics that you hold both as individuals or as a couple?

*LAMAR:* Yes, but no.

*MONTANA:* I agree. We have talked about a few things but nothing too much.

*THERAPIST:* Well this will be great then. A mentor of mine once said to me during my earlier training that has been extremely helpful and insightful. Couples must agree and align on the purposes of their relationship and the functioning of many things. When they do not, then problems can arise. Can you tell me what some of the values are that you have spoken about previously?

*MONTANA:* We have spoken about kids and how we like to spend our time together after work.

*THERAPIST:* This is great! What did you all say to each other about it and how did the conversation go?

*LAMAR:* We brought up the question about kids on the first date and we both agreed that we wanted them.

*MONTANA:* Yeah we did. I thought it was nice to see that he knew what he wanted and that we both wanted the same thing. There was not much more conversation about children after that with the exception of when we would try.

*THERAPIST:* Great! Thanks for sharing this. Could I inquire about the "time spent" conversation?

*LAMAR:* Yes. I don't like to waste time and spending that time with people that are my crew is very important. Montana and I make plans so that we can experience most of the things we do together.

*MONTANA:* Yeah, we plan out our time together pretty well. There are a few things that we could do less of but I agree with how we plan because it is important to Lamar and I do not mind putting in that effort.

*THERAPIST:* Thank you for this! One last question before we go into the values conversation. How did or do you know that you all agree and align with these values you have spoken about?

*MONTANA:* That is a good question. I think it's because when these topics come up, we don't have arguments about them. What do you think Lamar?

*LAMAR:* I agree. When we agree on things, we don't typically argue.

*THERAPIST:* This makes sense to me. Let's shift into the values alignment conversation if you don't mind. I have a list of values that I would like to through and explore if you all are in agreement or alignment in them. These values that I name are not exhaustive but have a major influence on intimate relationships. They are communication, sex, cleaning, family, money, intimate relationships, disagreements, dependency, independence, autonomy, and food.

Note: The therapist hands both Lamar and Montana a sheet of paper with the word "values" in the middle, and each of their names listed on either side of the word "values." Below the word "values" were a list of the said values (see Appendix A).

*THERAPIST:* Let's go through each of these and see your individual philosophy on them and if they align. If you both have divergent opinions and thoughts, we can talk through if you need to have them in agreement or alignment and/or the potential impact these things might have on your relationship.

Lamar and Montana revealed a great deal of overlap and agreement on the values presented by the therapist and had one area that did not and that had an impact on their relationship. They had differing views/philosophies on sex. The dialogue on this is below.

*THERAPIST:* So you all have different thoughts about sex. Montana, you stated that sex is important in the relationship but experience it more as exploration and expansion. You stated that you wish you could have more sexual openness with your husband. Lamar, you stated that sex is also important as it is an essential way of relating to your wife in a way that no other person can and that you do not like exploring sexual intimacy. Am I stating this correctly?

*LAMAR AND MONTANA:* Yes.

| | |
|---|---|
| *THERAPIST:* | Great. What do you make of this? Is having a different understanding or value of sex an impact for you all? |
| *LAMAR AND MONTANA:* | Yes. |
| *MONTANA:* | I don't think it's a big deal, but I sometimes believe Lamar is a little restrictive on what we do and how he responds to the things I would want to try. |
| *THERAPISTS:* | Lamar, do you have thoughts on what Montana stated? |
| *LAMAR:* | No, I agree. |
| *THERAPIST:* | Alright, what has gotten in the way of sharing this with each other? |
| *LAMAR:* | Well it's coming up now because you asked about it and we normally do not talk about sex in this way. |
| *THERAPIST:* | Mmmhmm. |
| *MONTANA:* | (turns toward Lamar) I feel like it is hard for you to hear some of the things I want to see happen in our sex life. I mean, it's hard for me also but people just typically go around talking about sex and what they want to do all the time right? I mean, it's a private issue. |
| *THERAPIST:* | Yes, sex and sexuality are personal and relational topics, but there is stigma locked in about how we value sex, its role in relationships, and even how we decide to talk (or not talk) about it. Part of the process in highlighting values that are divergent is affirming that relationships come in all sorts of arrangements and you all have the flexibility to be connected sexually in the way that works for you all. There is no wrong, what only works for you. |

Lamar and Montana have stumbled into a space that is often undiscovered by many therapists working with couples and intimate relationships. The alignment of values and where they clash are often presented as "communication issues," "trouble in fighting" and to borrow a term from the Gottman method (Gottman & Gottman, 2013), "unresolvable or perpetual problems." The issue is that their values are misaligned, and they are stuck on the content of what they are attempting to speak about. In addition, issues such as sexuality, sexual orientation, sexual roles, and pleasure connected to intimacy are surface level in conversation. The identification of a person's "Love Language"

(Chapman, 2009) is often helpful for folx to start visualizing the way they wish to show affection and how they can demonstrate a preferred form of affection for their partner(s); however, the conversation and understanding of where these values come are unspoken about. The values exercise and sheet (appendix) are extremely helpful to therapists and relationships that require an expansive view and understanding of how they operate, how their partner(s) operate, and the ways in which they have freedom to be aligned and/or develop a process that supports meeting the needs of their partner(s).

## Values—Clinical Application Exercises

### *Implementing Values Alignment in Your Practice*

#### *The Values Worksheet and Values Alignment Process*

Unlike surface preference discussions, MRT's Values work creates insight to core beliefs that shape relational dynamics. Begin by distinguishing between inherited values and chosen values based on the values worksheet (Appendix A). Once that has been completed, the Values Alignment process can begin as detailed below.

#### *Values Alignment Setup*

##### *Materials Needed*

- Values Worksheet (see Appendix A)
- Colored markers (assorted colors for each partner)
- Large paper for mapping
- Post-it notes for fluid exploration

#### *The Values Interview Protocol*

Begin with individual exploration before couple's work:

##### *Individual Session Questions*

1. "If your relationship were a refuge, what would be sacred there?"
2. "What values would you die defending? Which would you release to save the relationship?"
3. "When you imagine your partnership five years from now, what values are still important and present?"
4. "What values did your family teach? Which serve you, which harm you?"

*Facilitation Technique: The Values Constellation*

Rather than listing values, create a living constellation:

1 **Core Values** (center): nonnegotiable, identity-defining
2 **Orbiting Values** (middle ring): important but flexible
3 **Peripheral Values** (outer ring): preferences that could shift
4 **Banished Values** (outside the circles): values to actively reject

Have partners create individual constellations, then overlay them to see alignment and tension points.

*Clinical Interventions*

The Values Conflict Protocol:

1 **Name without Shame**: "You value security, they value adventure. Neither is wrong."
2 **Explore the Why**: "What does security mean to you? What experiences shaped this need?"
3 **Find the Fear**: "What terrifies you about their value? What threatens you about yours?"
4 **Seek the Bridge**: "How might security and adventure coexist? Where are they already?"
5 **Create Experiments**: "What if we tried living your value this week, theirs next week?"

The Sexual Values Conversation:

Therapist: "Let's talk about what you value sexually. Not what you do, but why you what you do."

- Pleasure as priority versus pleasure as privilege
- Sex as connection versus sex as release
- Monogamy as safety versus monogamy as constraint
- Bodies as temples versus bodies as playgrounds

*Common Clinical Stumbling Blocks*

**When Clients Say**: "We value the same things but still fight."
**MRT Response**: "Same words, different definitions. When you say 'family,' what do you mean? When they say it, what do they mean? It is important to confirm the working definitions that everyone holds."
**When Clients Say**: "Their values are just wrong."

**MRT Response**: "Values aren't wrong, they're stories about what may tether us to a purpose and organize our relationships. What story is their value telling? What danger is it protecting against?"

### Exercises and Discussion Questions

1. Lamar and Montana discovered misaligned values around sexuality. How do you create safety for couples to explore sexual values that may challenge religious, cultural, or family teachings? What is your role when values conflict with institutional beliefs?
2. Black Queer relationships are described as consistently discussing and managing values due to lived experiences of oppression. How can you help other couples develop this same skill set for ongoing values negotiation?
3. This chapter suggests moving beyond "Love Languages" to deeper values exploration. How might surface-level relationship tools inadvertently avoid the more challenging but necessary conversations about fundamental values?
4. How do you help clients distinguish between values that are authentically theirs versus those inherited from family, culture, or religion? What does values-based authenticity look like in practice?

# 7 Power and the Power Analysis

A working definition for the word of power I would like to offer you is "The ability or capacity to do something or act in a particular way." This definition will be a mutual understanding of how this chapter on power is framed and how you can understand how it is applied. Power is a topic that is often not spoken about directly and often is not noticeable unless there is an absence of it. Families and intimate relationships are notorious for showing up in our therapy rooms and offices with conflicts about dishes, mealtimes, homework not being done, disrespectful conversations, and a lack of agreement on how to proceed in solving problems. This is the content; however, the process of the dynamic is a power struggle.

Knowledge about power is elusive yet visible in society. We speak about power in our schools found in subjects such as Politics, Social Studies, and other topics regarding governance. Knowledge of power is seen in various social movements and community advocacy that seek to mobile collectively the shared power for social change. Families are also sources of knowledge regarding power where lessons are ingrained from early ages about authority, permission, consent, and abilities to make decisions.

Black families pass on knowledge about power early on as means to inform and protect their family unit. These are found in the direct and matter of fact conversations relating police presence/encounters via "the talk" and the encouragement needed to keep one's head down and do well in school by avoiding racial and ethnic bias in academic spaces.

Alongside Black families, the Queer community is just as knowledgeable about power and how it is used against them. Social visibility of Queer people has come about from mobilizing shared resources to promote change within society; much of this resistance lives in the philosophy of pride marches which stand for the pushback against oppression toward the LGBTQ community.

Power in Western cultures has been professed to come about through individual effort and exceptional talent where in perhaps a few cases this is true. The unspoken truth is that power often rests with others due to the resources that they possess, which have been passed down by generations previously. The previous generations often profited from the oppression of others and

DOI: 10.4324/9781032725987-7

consolidation of power. Conversations about power are missing on purpose within our larger communities. If we were to have truthful and participatory dialogue about power, it would mean that there is an acknowledgment of how our societies work and those who hold and maintain power by inequitable means would lose that power.

Many times, we are not taught how to speak about power, how to share it in relationships, and the benefits of power sharing which result in power struggles. In these power struggles, members of the relational unit either seek to keep the power for themselves as it helps them remain in control and maintain making decisions or seek ways to regain or reclaim power as they are disenfranchised. These positions leave people feeling unfulfilled, lonely, helpless, and listless; fueling distance between them with each disagreement becomes increasingly entrenched in the struggle. Ironically, we lack comprehensive language about power in relationships as they are connected to our society as stated above.

Black Queer relationships are no stranger to issues of power as these identities (Black, Queer) often are lacking in power as compared White heterosexual cisgendered individuals. The prevalence of Double Consciousness (Du Bois, 2022) burns bright. Black Queer folx have learned to thrive in times where and when they lacked power to directly change their oppressive environment. This resiliency has prompted them to learn how to not replicate harmful relational patterns that limit how power transfers from one person to another or balances the power in said relationship(s).

The act of sharing power requires all parties to be willing to collaborate in finding a particular formula or percentage of power that person has which allows for a maximum amount of agency and flexibility. This can be better named as a Power Analysis. In this process of collaboration, folx let go of their need to make decisions based on what they think or what is best for them individually. They open themselves up to hear what the other relational unit(s) have to say and validates their standpoint. Likewise, they make room to share their needs and be validated in that said need and the connecting context they share. This process of reciprocity and open dialogue assists the relational unit in developing a truly multirelational and multidimensional agreement to avoid power struggles.

Black Queer relationships know this dance of power sharing. They have been choreographing it for centuries. In traditional relationships, sexual roles are based on traditional views of sex. That is cis men are more active and dominant (top) than their cis female partners and said cis female partners are to be submissive and receive (bottom). Queer relationships, specifically in Black men, have greater levels of satisfaction due to the presence of love and their flexibility in relationships (Edwards, 2016). A source of this flexibility is in their sexual roles; either accepting some of the dyadic division of sexual intercourse in traditional relationships or allowing for free choice in their sexual experience. In a two-person relationship, one partner will top, and the other will bottom and continue with this arrangement as it works for them. Perhaps in another two-person relationship, there will be two tops, and they invite a third to be their bottom. And in other relational agreements of a two-person relationship, they are both bottoms and satisfy each other with the use of toys or invite another to play the role of a top. A further arrangement in a two-person relationship is that both partners are versatile (meaning the freely oscillate and choose between top, bottom, or side) and can satisfy any role they choose to. Perhaps they are sides where penetration is not the focus and sexual gratification comes from other activities and engagements (kissing, touching, mutual masturbation, and toys). All these scenarios and even more lead to power being shared within the sexual relationship. Of course, it should be noted that Black Queer relationships are not a monolith, and you will find relationships that are Black and Queer but have trouble sharing power, specifically in sexual experiences.

To further ground the understanding of power and how to conduct a Power Analysis, we will return to the case of Lamar and Montana who are discussing how decision-making around shared activities that involved nonpreferred events were rooted in a power struggle and how the use of a power analysis and the subsequent sharing of power helped bring balance to the relationship.

Session opening

*LAMAR:* Hey Dr. I have something on my mind that I want to discuss today.

*THERAPIST:* Awesome. Is this something that Montana knows about?

*LAMAR:* Yes, we spoke about it in the car coming over. It is about how we spend time doing activities that I like but Montana does not.

*THERAPIST:* Okay. That sounds like a good place to begin. Are you able to check in with Montana about her desire to address this issue? Lamar turns to Montana

*LAMAR:* Are you cool with us talking about what you discussed in the car about you coming skiing?

*MONTANA:* Yep.

*THERAPIST:* Alright, Lamar, can you share what is on your mind?

*LAMAR:* Sure. So, we have been making progress in therapy and our communication has gotten better but we keep hitting a wall about time spent.

*THERAPIST:* How so?

*LAMAR:* Well generally if we are spending time together doing something that we both want to do, going out with common friends, seeing family or out for a date, we do not have issues. However, when we are supposed to do something that is more geared toward what I like to do, it is apparent that Montana does not want to be there. Half of the time it takes such an effort to get her there and when she is there, there is no joy or happiness. It kills me."

*THERAPIST:* Thank you for sharing that Lamar. I am wondering if we can hear from Montana regarding her viewpoint.

*LAMAR:* Go right ahead.

*THERAPIST:* Montana, what is your understanding about this issue that Lamar brought up? I would like to know what your perspective is.

*MONTANA:* Well, he is correct. I really do try and like the things he likes but I feel like we are completely opposites about everything. I really do attempt but it is just awful. It brings down the mood and I feel like it is a big issue in our relationship.

*THERAPIST:* Thank you both for sharing this. My first question for you all is what attempts have you made at solving this problem?

*LAMAR:* We try to talk about it but it usually goes south and we get into an argument.

Therapist gestures to Montana to share

*MONTANA:* Yeah, the conversations usually go nowhere. I am beginning to think this will always be an issue that we cannot solve.

*THERAPIST:* Lamar, I am wondering what is important to you about the decision-making process between you two regarding these activities.

*LAMAR:* It is important because couples need to spend time together right? How else do they bond?

*THERAPIST:* That is absolutely true but also somewhat of common knowledge for all relationships. For you, however in this intimate relationship, what is important in spending that time or even in the process of deciding what to do?

(A few seconds pause)

*LAMAR:* It feels as if she does not want to spend time with me and the act of coming to an agreement is too much for her. It is like I cannot ask her for anything.

Power is something that is extremely elusive in the relationship between Lamar and Montana. They are conflicted in part with how and when they spend time together, which is true; however, the decision-making process and who is allowed to "call the shots" is the larger issue here. The couple mentioned this conflict in session to address a particular hurt that was present for Lamar and named Montana's decision to not take part in the conversation (and to designate it as an argument they will never solve) as a source of disconnection. Utilizing a power analysis is bringing form to function where overt and covert rules and dynamics of a system shape responses and the positionality of people to one another. In this example, the therapist uses the power analysis to find out who has power, where they use it (or do not), how it is used, and when they may choose to wield this energy. In this case, Montana has power to make herself available to Lamar in the capacity that he wishes for her to be and to choose how she can be present in the way that she would like. In addition, Montana's vulnerability stays hidden in this dynamic as she makes the decision to either be present or find a way to connect with Lamar in his preferred activity or move away from it.

It is also important to highlight that in this transcript, Montana does have the right to rebuff Lamar for his request in her taking part in her nonpreferred activity. This example may also be heightened as it may present itself as Montana making herself available to Lamar solely based on her sex and gender which is oppressive and one directional. Conducting a power analysis and examining how and where power is used should not be used to reinforce (or create) unhealthy dynamics or further oppression. The power analysis and conversation regarding power should be used with the consent of the relationship and seek to provide people the room to be expansive in their agreements and how they can make themselves available and vulnerable to one another. The congestion of power in relationships may lead to unhealthy relationship dynamics such as pursuer-distancer (Betchen, 2013), fear and shame (Epstein & Falconier, 2017), or demand-withdraw (Eldridge & Christensen, 2002). Many major models have interventions that address these dynamics, but most do not support therapists to create additional awareness as to how power is held.

Power lives differently within many relationships of color. In Black Queer relationships, there may be more freedom to explore these issues and acceptance for you to mention this. However, in other populations, there may be strong resistance to reorganizing their relationship dynamics to accommodate how power is assessed. Therapists who treat diverse clients who have strong religious or spiritual beliefs should be aware that the client system convictions may mandate that power flows in predetermined ways. The use of the power analysis is and should be respectful or where and how people have consented into roles. First, the therapist should examine if the folx in the relationship are open to challenging the norms of their spiritual/religious and/or cultural norms and that there is safety present in doing so. Second, the therapist should not assume that because they are religious/spiritual or align to a specific cultural norm that there is oppression present. It is the responsibility of the therapist to be curious about the relationship and inquire where they are situated. A full overview of the Power Analysis can be found in Appendices C and D.

While the transcript of the client session covered only the presence of a power imbalance and ways to expand and/or share power in the relationship, the full explanation of the Power Analysis will be shared now. It is important to know that some client systems may be resistant to identifying and agreeing that there are power imbalances present in the relationship. Therapists should take care to support their clients in understanding that community equity, be it in our homes, our extended families, our intimate relationships, or greater ecological surroundings, only strengthens what we have and increases the ability for folx to be responsible and accountable to themselves and each other.

The Power Analysis begins with a simple question, "Who is running things?" Then we dig deeper and ask, "Where does their power come from? Is it their money, their gender, and their voice that fills the room?" We then map it out to gain a better understanding of the dynamics in the relationship that will assist us in promoting conversations around the balancing of power and the sharing of power.

When mapping the power in the system, we create an understanding of the sources of power in the relationship, their power sources, and other players that have an impact on the system (Appendix C and D contain a walkthrough). To analyze the power dynamics in the map, the therapist should list the places/sources of power and denote the corresponding symbols to their charge (Taking power—utilizing a "+" symbol; Shared power—utilizing an "=" symbol; and Power taken—utilizing a "–"symbol). Following the analysis of power, the balancing of power occurs with therapist support. In balancing power, a proper critique of domination, if present, must be done. "Dominance. Control. These things the unjust seek most of all. And so, it is the duty of the just to defy dominance and to challenge control" (Fanney, 2005). As such if the relationship structure is set to be one of control over and without consent of so, the system will need to be challenged to abandon this relationship and is present as a barrier to the flow of power in a multidirectional manner. Once the domination has been removed, the client system can come together and determine how they desire to realign their structure and make decisions that are respectful of each other while supporting their agency. This is called collective agency. Once the system can exercise their collective agency, they will be able to articulate their own responsibility and accountability, which is the last sub-step of the Power Balancing intervention. Intimate relationships that are embedded with responsibility allow for individual members to have control over their actions, voice their concerns, exercise their agency to make requests of the other(s) and show up in their fullest capacity when possible, and share when they are unable to. Intimate relationships that are imbued with accountability create opportunities for individual members to own the container of themselves, that is, their bodies, body-minds, intellect, desire, affection, and presence to form and maintain appropriate boundaries and connections. In addition, intimate relationships where all members of that system enact both responsibility and accountability on the individual and system level create effective structures that flow with the ability to nurture health relational dynamics, namely, safety, autonomy, and determination.

The last step of the Power Analysis is the sharing of Power. This step unfolds in three actions, each building on the last. The act of sharing power ensures that the client system has a pathway of moving power equitably and responsibly between all people and can be flexible in mobilizing resources and decision-making, increasing their ability to survive problems and thrive in their victories. The first step necessary to share power is to engage in Community Care. The relational systems that we are bound by often need care and have been overshadowed by notions of self-care. The push for the care of self or self-care, specifically as therapists, is important as it prevents elements of compassion fatigue and affirming rest within our profession; however, it is focused only on the individual and misses key aspects of care and how we share power. Care of the community we exist in, which includes relationships, allows for multidirectional avenues of support, affection, communication, sharing of resources, and verbalization of priorities. Through these vital conversations and connections, we can name the ways we need help and the ways we can provide help, and the production of that help and support come by power (i.e., the act of making something come to fruition). The second sub-step is Inclusivity. While Community Care is about caring for the community or relational unit(s) we utilize this work with, the *who* we include is important. The sharing of power with the aim to include others assists in creating normative experiences that we will and should include others in the consideration of holding and increasing the flow of power. This point is best seen with the application of this model in family intervention or in its use with a throuple or other intimate relationship constellation with more than two folx. While families should organize in ways that allow them to function in a way that prioritizes their needs, too strong of hierarchies and boundaries resulting in the distance between parents and children or other family members such as grandparents to other subsystems may need more power in order to either be more active in the system or move through their own stage of human/family development. Likewise, the inclusivity of who is consulted with in the movement of power in polyamorous relationships is extremely important. A relationship with three people will find themselves best served when everyone in that system is aware of where and how power was moved and to who(m).

The last sub-step of sharing of Power is Justice. The movement and sharing of power should be rooted in regard that when people recognize that power has been denied to them or that we keep power for the purpose of self-interest, we remove opportunities to demonstrate love and respect to those to which we are connected. Justice in relationships and in power sharing seeks to ensure that there should always be consideration and action to be right in relationship with another.

The work of Balancing and Sharing of power within relationships is often harder than most people care to admit. The movement of power away from a person who may have held power in either selfish or egocentric manners may prompt feeling of loss and grief, and in some cases, extreme vulnerability. These feelings are difficult and some folx may be averse or avoidant in addressing them and present as extremely resistant or defensive. Balancing and Sharing of Power should be coupled with safety for the client system and full of reminders of what can be realized on the other side of realignment.

## Power Analysis—Clinical Application

### *Implementing the Power Analysis in Your Practice*

#### *Preparing for Conversations Regarding Power*

Power discussions trigger defenses. Prepare clients by normalizing power dynamics.

Therapist introduction to the conversation: "Every relationship has power dynamics. The question is not whether power exists, but whether it is acknowledged and shared. Today we map power not to judge one another but to understand the function and role it plays."

#### *The Power Mapping Process*

**Step 1: Identify Power Sources**—Use the Power Mapping Worksheet (Appendix D) with these categories:

- Money/wealth (Who controls money?)
- Mental health (Who manages feelings and presence of mental health issues?)
- Sexuality (Who initiates? Who refuses?)
- Sexual position (Which positions and roles decided or enacted?)
- Community (Who determines friendships? Who determines how supports are accessed)
- Domestic (Who decides home matters?)
- Gender presentation (Who decides which presentations are acceptable?)
- Family of origin (Who decided which people are included as family?)
- Other sources of power which are free to be added based on the needs of the client system.

**Step 2: Map Current Distribution**—For each source, mark for each person:

- (+) I hold this power.
- (−) They hold this power.
- (=) We share this power.
- (?) Unclear who holds this power.

**Step 3: Analyze the Pattern**—Questions for exploration:

- "Where does power concentrate?"
- "Which power distributions were chosen? Which were assumed?"
- "How does external oppression shape internal power dynamics?"
- "Where does power flow? Where does it stagnate?"

*Clinical Interventions*

***The Power Exchange Experiment***

Prompt: "What if we switched who holds what for one week?"

Design specific exchanges for the client system. Below are examples:

- Person who usually initiates sex must wait to be approached.
- Person who manages money hands over financial decisions.
- Person who plans social events steps back.
- The person who normally occupies the dominate role in sex becomes submissive.

Process the discomfort, fear, and surprise that arise when these prompts are discussed.

***The Power Sharing Process***

Moving from Power-Over to Power-With:

1 **Identify One Hoarded Power**: "I realize I control all our social plans."
2 **Explore the Why**: "I fear if I don't, we'll be isolated."
3 **Name the Impact**: "This leaves you feeling unheard about our social life."
4 **Design the Share**: "What if we alternate monthly who plans?"
5 **Create Accountability**: "How will we know if I'm taking power back?"

*Addressing Power in Black Queer Relationships*

Special considerations for therapists to consider asking their client systems: "In a world that denies you power everywhere, how do you share it at home?"

Explore these examples:

- How racism creates power hoarding as survival
- How homophobia shapes sexual power dynamics
- How both partners may feel simultaneously powerful and powerless
- The difference between power taken by society and power given to partner

*Common Clinical Challenges*

**Challenge**: "Talking about power feels like keeping score."
**MRT Response**: "Scorekeeping is language that limits our options. When we map out power and understand why it is held, informed decisions about how it is shared can be made."
**Challenge**: "They don't want to share power in [specific area]"
**MRT Response**: "Let's unpack what they may lose if it was shared. Power hoarding often comes from powerlessness elsewhere. Where else do they lack control?"

## Exercises and Discussion Questions

1 This chapter states that conversations about power are "missing on purpose" in Western culture. How do you overcome client resistance to discussing power when they have been socialized to avoid these conversations? What is your strategy for making power visible without creating defensiveness?
2 Using the Power Analysis framework (Appendices C and D), conduct a power mapping of a current couple or family you are working with. What sources of power do you identify, and how might balancing these powers change their dynamics?
3 The concept of "collective agency" is presented as essential for healthy relationships. How do you help clients move from individual decision-making to collaborative power sharing? What obstacles typically arise?
4 Black Queer relationships are noted for their flexibility in sexual roles as an example of power sharing. How can you help clients expand their understanding of power beyond traditional gender roles across all areas of their relationship?
5 This chapter warns against using power analysis to reinforce oppression or create unhealthy dynamics. How do you ensure that power sharing conversations genuinely increase equity rather than simply redistributing control?
6 "Justice in relationships" is presented as the last step of power sharing. How do you help clients understand and practice justice as an ongoing relational value rather than a one-time correction?

# 8 Liberation

A quote by bell hooks is a fitting opening to understand this tenet: "The moment we choose to love we begin to move against domination, against oppression. The moment we choose to love we begin to move toward freedom, to act in ways that liberate ourselves and others" (hooks, 1994). For this chapter and the next (Radical Emancipation), we will no longer explore the model via their sessions as their journey with Multidynamic Relational Therapy (MRT) became intensely personal. They did not give permission for those parts of the sessions to be utilized to explain MRT. It is also fitting as Chapters 9 and 10 are highly subjective to everyone. That is, the landing points of these interventions are based on each person's intersections. Kimberly Crenshaw's famous intersectionality framework (Crenshaw, 2019) provided a wonderful template to begin to understand how oppression impacts a person. Intersectionality is not just listing off identities that are oppressed or have power. We miss a vital point in not understanding the fullness of what Crenshaw requested us to comprehend. When an individual has a part of them that is subject to oppressive interactions, there are barriers that create hidden and unimaginable dynamics in folx accessing the things they want and need. Liberation according to MRT creates an environment where those hidden dynamics become visible and perhaps even tangible so that they can be confronted, tamed, and personally addressed.

The term "liberation" has been around for a while describing various social and physical movements and personal philosophies and the struggle for independence and autonomy. Much like the Black liberation movements, the psychology liberation movement and women's liberation movement, this model seeks to highlight the necessity of being free and freedom of individuals and communities to exist without oppression. The Black liberation movement (Carmichael, 1966) sought to create conditions for Black people to be free from the intellectual, physical, emotional, and financial bondage that limited their ability to move forward in motion within their own families and communities. The movement sought to create pathways for individuals to contextualize what opportunities that desired to create within their lives and produce both tangible and intangible outcomes that aligned with their

DOI: 10.4324/9781032725987-8

decision-making and not the limits placed on what they were told to do. The Black Liberation movement even used outward manifestations of appearance via clothing and fashion to show their freedom from oppression and departure from normative dress codes that focused on Eurocentric appeals and demands (Vargas, 2009). This fantastic fashion and outlandish use of color, texture, and patterns was not necessarily new for the Black community to use. During the late 1700s in now what is called the state of Louisiana in the United States, Creole women were forbidden to reveal their natural hair in public as it was seen as improper and offensive. This law was called Tignon's law (Ngandu-Kalenga Greensword, 2022). The Black and Brown women during this time found a way to survive by pushing back on the oppressive laws that sought to govern, monitor and criminalize their minds and bodies. The woman followed the law requiring them to hide their hair, but they found a way to challenge the narratives of oppression in the law by tying their hair in beautiful wraps which was seen to attract more attention and desire from others than before. The government at that time sought to suppress Black and biracial freed women and keep the hierarchy of white people higher than them and visually label who was free and/or connected to slavery.

The Women's suffrage movement was yet another example of liberation within communities of people. Women over the course of history have contributed to the advancement of society, yet they remained second-class citizens and many times property of their fathers of husband. Of course, there are historical accounts of women, specifically in African history, that are well revered for their power, resistance, leadership, and vision. Queen Nzinga Mbandi, once the leader of Angola, is known for her organization and strategic war time skills that lead her people, the Mbundu, to resist occupation by the Portuguese (Pantoja, 2020). She continues to be revered in as a skilled leader and one with a strong and sharp vision. Yaa Asantewaa, once queen of the Ashanti tribe, played a vital role as the leader who unified her tribe to push back against the British invasion of Ghana in spanning from the 1870s until 1900 (Brempong, 2000). While these efforts were not enough to prevent British occupation, Yaa ensured that her people did not lose connection with their culture and customs and fought to ensure that who they were did not fade away even when their home was stolen from them.

As was listed above in just those two examples, women have played pivotal roles to preserve their communities' power and identity in the face of fierce boundaries and suppression. While these movements were for all people, the Women's suffrage movement was for women. The pushback against the norms and cultural, religious, and community expectations for anyone who was a woman was great and threatened the social dynamics and fabrics of society, rightfully so. It is a shame that it was not enough for women to protest their absence of their power, but that men had to agree and validate this standpoint to actualize it. This movement sought to liberation women from a position of subordinate and without position to determine their own destinies.

Lastly, the liberation movement within psychology, also known as Liberation Psychology, is twofold. The first is its notion that therapeutic philosophy and treatment should and does transcend the traditional tenets of psychological intervention that pull from various critical theories that center people of color and other oppressed individuals (Comas-Díaz, 2020). The second notion is that the furthering of this framework relies on practitioners that execute methods that reflect the tenets of anti-oppression, freedom from bondage, restoration from collection amnesia, and disconnect by utilizing research methods such as participatory action research (a form of research that is community focused and ultimately returns ownership of the data and outcomes to the community that is being researched) (Kidd & Kral, 2005) and alternative expressions of emotions and being (e.g., Art therapies). Liberation Psychology was created and developed in Latin America with Ignacio Martin-Baro being credited with its creator.

MRT follows suit with these examples in history regarding liberation of the self and community. Within the MRT model, liberation is one of the last interventions in place, alongside Radical Emancipation, allowing for individuals to find a way to live their lives in the way they choose to and find individual freedom in their expression. Liberation allows individuals to determine, to their extent, how to exercise control over their minds, bodies, intellect, and spirit. The right to believe in their heart about the tenets of their freedom. The right to have autonomy of their bodies by wearing their hair in the way they choose, to carry a child or not, and to connect themselves sexually with others or not in the preferences of their mind. The right to believe and right about the philosophies of their freedom and have access to the information that compliments their lived experiences, and lastly to dream and plan their lives according to their own desires, safety, relationships, visions, and hear.

People of color and specifically Black people who may be LGBTQ+ have been fighting for years for autonomy over themselves and over their own decisions which include who they will love, commune, and even sleep with. These decisions have often been monitored and regulated by using faulty scientific theories of inferiority or magical thinking that make Black people both subhuman and superhuman at the same time (Mills, 2015). Yet, Black people within the LGBTQ+ communities have fought against this oppression and, despite the odds, have figured out how to live a life that does not necessarily rid one of said oppression, but gives yourself permission to seek out and display who you are unapologetically and authentically. This can be seen in its most vibrant form at Ballroom events and experiences. More about this influence will be shared in Chapter 11.

The previous steps/interventions from earlier in the book prepare the therapist to build on the work done with clients to give them a more substantive stage to continue their healing work that comes about from traumatic experiences that often extend from mismatched values, hidden expectations, unrealized wisdom, and a world that many times seeks conformity at the cost of the erasure of those who may be different. Special note: Liberation is not a one-time performance; it is a song that we return to finding new joy and expression. We are confronted with multiple problems which many of them are simply unsolvable as it would require a collective reset of our world and revisit what our joint purpose of humanity is (i.e., the need for money, work, discriminatory practices toward one another, etc.). Clients will come to a place where they are unable to solve the problem that brings them in; however, they choose joy. They choose connection. They choose freedom and they choose to be flexible and reflexive in their inner world. Think about for you, coming into an understanding about this model within the context of your own life. How many times do you think you would come, or at least desire, to a place of liberation? Continued instances of liberation are contagious and give folx an opportunity to create new flexible possibilities toward their view of life and the relationships that they keep.

We as therapists should seek to give our clients, clients in intimate relationships, and client families substantive frameworks to find healing that transcends verbal processing and traditional linear Eurocentric ways of being. There has been much value in the lessons and tenets of personal tenacity and determination that were found in many of the philosophies and leadership skills of the people mentioned earlier in this chapter. Much of what has made their pathways of liberation successful is the very things that they sought to protect from erasure due to laws and racism, and found ways to preserve and transform into something more magnificent and precious than before.

## Liberation—Clinical Application

### *Understanding Liberation in the Therapy Room*

Liberation is not a one-time occurrence according to the model and in lived experiences. It is an ongoing practice of choosing freedom of expression over constraint. In MRT, we facilitate liberation by helping client systems identify where oppression lives in their relationships and support them to prioritize how to live authentically within their bodies and minds.

### *Preliberation Assessment*

Before diving into liberation work, assess readiness within the system by inquiring about:

- Have societal expectations been identified and managed appropriately?
- Are values defined, clarified, consented to, and aligned?
- Has power been mapped within the system and have there been opportunities to create a template for sharing power?

- Is there sufficient safety to challenge deep ingrained narratives that may prevent moving forward?

## *The Liberation Process*

### *Phase 1: Identifying Internalized Oppression*

"Where does oppression live in your love or your body?"

Through targeted conversations and questions, we can help clients recognize:

- Internalized homophobia ("We can't be too gay in public.")
- Internalized racism ("We need to be respectable.")
- Internalized sexism ("Someone has to be the 'man'.")
- Internalized classism ("We're not successful enough to matter.")

### *Phase 2: Tracing the Source*

"Whose voice tells you that you're too much? Not enough?"

Map the journey:

- The origin of the message sourced
- How it came to be reinforced and ingrained
- Current spaces that this oppression or narrative of oppression exists
- The cost it has to the relationship (to oneself and/or others)

### *Phase 3: Choosing Resistance*

"What would a small rebellion of freedom look and feel like?"

Encourage client systems to start small while considering safety issues. Examples of this small resistance could look like:

- Hold hands in public.
- Correct someone who misgenders your partner.
- Wear something that is congruent with your identity.
- Say no to family expectations that may cause you harm.

## *Clinical Interventions*

*Below are interventions, ideas, language, and guiding exercises to assist client systems on how to navigate the process of liberation within their lives and in the therapy room. Clinicians have the ability to use one or all of these.*

*The Liberation Inventory*

Have client systems list:

1 Two to three ways oppression impacts their relationship
2 Two to three ways they already resist against
3 Three to four rebellions they daydream about as possibilities (even if it feels)
4 One rebellion they are willing to try this week, month, or year

*The Joy Practice*

Experiences of oppression make it extremely difficult to feel and hold onto joy. When people face consistent and constant invalidation and opposition to who they are, it can feel unsafe to express their true selves. This can make joy fleeting, fragile, or just out of reach. Practicing joy can be an act of resistance by giving yourself full permission to exist when the world tells you otherwise. Choosing to nurture light and delight creates an opportunity to reclaim space to be whole and authentic.

Weekly joy assignments:

- Dance in your kitchen.
- Make love in daylight.
- Laugh too loudly.
- Take up space.

*The Grief Process*

The liberation process often includes grief and loss. It is important to recognize that promotion of an authentic expression of self may create a separation of a person from their known community. These themes or types of grief and loss that may be present:

- Grieving safety in conformity
- Mourning the loss family acceptance, visibility, and belonging
- Releasing approval addiction
- Letting go of "normal" and comforts associated with being grouped with a majority

Hold space for this grief without rushing toward "positivity" or resolution which may dilute the meaning making process for individuals.

*Common Clinical Challenges*

**Challenge**: "Promoting liberation feels selfish when others are suffering."
**MRT Response**: "Liberation is systemic and collective. Your individual freedom impacts and influences others. By freeing yourself, you show others that this is possible. Your joy won't diminish others' pain. It helps illuminate a path for others."
**Challenge**: "We'll lose everything if we embrace who we truly are."
**MRT Response**: "You very well might lose some things. But what are you losing by hiding? Is it worth it to you to be congruent? If so, let's grieve what you might lose and celebrate what you all will gain."

*Liberation Homework*

*Client systems can benefit from structured homework outside of sessions to help practice the process of liberation. Therapists should remember that practicing these interventions in session prior to being assigned homework supports successful completion of the work and clarifies questions.*

## Week 1: Oppression Inventory

- Document daily moments of shrinking.
- Notice body sensations when conforming.
- Track energy after code-switching.

## Week 2: Micro-Rebellions

- One tiny rebellion against a restricting idea daily.
- Document feelings before/during/after.
- Share with partner each evening.

## Week 3: Joy Practice

- Schedule three joy moments.
- Do one thing "too much."
- Celebrate without apology.

**Exercises and Discussion Questions**

1. Liberation is described as "not a one-time performance but a song we return to." How do you help clients understand liberation as an ongoing process rather than a destination? What does the maintenance of liberation look like in therapeutic practice?
2. This chapter emphasizes that liberation allows individuals to "determine how to exercise control over their minds, bodies, intellect and spirit." How do you support clients in reclaiming autonomy over areas where they've been systematically disempowered?
3. Historical examples like Tignon's law demonstrate how oppressed communities transformed restrictions into expressions of resistance and beauty. How can you help clients reframe their current constraints as opportunities for creative liberation?
4. This chapter notes that some problems are "simply unsolvable" due to systemic issues, yet clients can still "choose joy, connection, and freedom." How do you help clients find liberation within unchanged oppressive circumstances without promoting complacency?

# 9 Radical Emancipation

Audre Lorde states, "Without community there is no liberation, only the most vulnerable and temporary armistice between individual and her oppression" (Lorde, 1984, p. 112). This quote is fitting for this chapter and allows you to understand how the individual work of one person is connected to the larger groups of others.

Emancipation can be defined as the fact or process of being set free from legal, social, or political restrictions with the etymology coming from a Latin word combining the prefix e-, meaning "away," and *mancipare*, meaning "to transfer ownership of" (Merriam-Webster, n.d.). When we hear this word, there are often two references that come to mind. The first is the emancipation process for young adults (under 18 but generally no younger than 14 in many places) who seek approval from the court system to free themselves from the mandatory dynamic of a parent(s) having authority and control over their child's decisions and trajectory. The other reference is the Emancipation Proclamation, which is the executive order written by Abraham Lincoln requiring all states to free their slaves. In both references, there are some identical tenets being that of release and that of freedom. Emancipation requires that a person or people be in a condition of subjection. This subjection is not always one of a "negative" context, but it often is. Those who are subjected have been treated unfairly, unjustly, and/or without recourse to have a sense of autonomy. Their ability to make informed or even ill-informed decisions are compromised, scrutinized, and held with someone else usually who has more power than they do and power over them. Emancipation also requires freedom to be on the other side lest someone be released into a lesser degree of freedom which can be argued that is not emancipation.

Radical Emancipation within the confines of MRT creates a continual stance of change within the relationships of the individual or system that has been liberated. They build on the work from the previous sections/interventions to create a way of being that assists them in putting form into the fashion of their desires and a place where they are free from oppression and interference. They can be clear on the vision of their lives and who they want to be connected to and the shape and composition of their partners and communities. It is a

DOI: 10.4324/9781032725987-9

profound relationship shifting position to be in and is often contagious. Change within systemic intervention (which this author encourages all practitioners to be trained in and practice) is layered and the goal is to create conditions for third-order change (McDowell et al., 2019). First-order change (Watzlawick et al., 2011) which can be found within individual, older models of therapy such as psychodynamic theory, cognitive-behavioral therapy (CBT), and dialectical behavioral therapy (DBT) focuses on the change of thinking and/or behavioral shifts that decrease some psychic distress. Second-order change (Davey et al., 2012) which can be found in the majority of systemic/family/couples-based models of therapy focuses on changing the relationship between individuals in the system and takes on more complex issues and dynamics as the "space between them" is where problems may be created and/or maintained. Teresa McDowell, Carmen Knudson-Martin, and J. Maria Bermudez (McDowell et al., 2019) introduced the concept of third-order change in their text Socioculturally *Attuned Family Therapy*. The authors expertly describe the need for clinicians to support their clients to go above and beyond the traditional paradigm of change in relationships. They argued that change is best served when we empower folx within systemic interventions and interactions and support them to make this change within their communities, be in their home, family, friends, places of worship, or geographical location (McDowell et al., 2019).

Radical Emancipation goes beyond the traditional ideas of change and nests it within a series of changes both within the individual and outside into their relationships. The individual that enables Radical Emancipation does so in the presence of new types of relationships that are the materialized spaces and visions of liberation. The relationships are no longer subject to faulty or pressurized societal expectations that were forced upon them. The relationship has created an avenue where their values are aligned and reflect who they wish to be in the world and originate from their intimate conversations, collaboration and creation. The relationships balance power between themselves to share in the ability to make change within their system and are grounded in mutuality, compassion, and respect. What is interesting about this state of relational being and stance is that it creates new types of communities to exist within. Black Queer relationships have long lived outside of the bounds of what was considered normal, yet they existed and even preserved. To be a Black Queer individual meant that your race was always a determining factor of how you were/are treated and subject to discrimination based on your skin color. And at the same time, your sexuality was/is scrutinized as an afront to nature and departed from religious standards of what a person should be. There are even more conditions that are placed on these individuals that do not extend from religious oppression or racism reasoning. Black Queer people found that they were not accepted in many of the circles that purported to be about accepting of said identity (i.e., Black Queer people being accepted in Black communities) and were stuck in a dynamic where limited belonging existed. Black Queer folx casted off the confines of that dynamic to create a realization of relationships that were grounded in who they were and what they wanted in the world despite what laws and attitudes prescribed about them and their relational connections. Research shows that Black Gay men have higher relationship satisfaction despite many of the challenges that they endure (Shepler et al., 2021; Edwards, 2016). This challenges norms that Queer relationships are unable to form lasting bonds of closeness and satisfaction, and this satisfaction is linked to their ability to thrive despite the pressures and stress they experience.

Traditional therapeutic models, however well-intentioned, were created within systems that rarely acknowledged how racism, homophobia, and other oppression impact the individual and shape relational dynamics. They offer interventions for "communication problems" and individual pathology without addressing how issues such as code-switching exhaustion impacts emotional availability or treat "sexual dysfunction" without considering how internalized shame from religious trauma affects desire and connection with oneself. These models assume a neutral playing field that simply does not exist for communities under siege. MRT brings this lived wisdom of resistance into therapeutic practice through a clinical framework, transforming what Black Queer folx have always known as an essential truth. Personal healing and political liberation are inseparable sides of the same freedom that are intertwined.

Radical Emancipation is not necessarily a new idea as it has existed within this community for years. MRT brings it to the mainstream within the world of psychotherapy in hopes that this penultimate piece of resistance and reform can revolutionize how people are able to create meaningful relationships that come from the autonomy of their humanity which is a right for all. Radical Emancipation can be the fourth- order change that transforms how therapy shifts communities into healthy relationships.

## Implementing Radical Emancipation in Your Practice

### *Recognizing Readiness for Radical Emancipation*

Not every client system reaches Radical Emancipation, which is okay. Not reaching Radical Emancipation is not indicative of a poor outcome of therapy within MRT. Many times, client systems will continue to evolve and change after our time with them. However, should individuals present as willing to engage in the process of Radical Emancipation, therapists can assess readiness indicators such as:

- Consistent liberation practices that are internalized and have become a part of daily life

- Internalized oppression significantly reduced evidenced by decreased symptomology connected to said oppression
- Power flows freely between partners and family members
- Values are consented to, aligned, and alive
- Societal expectations consciously chosen, rejected, or modified
- Client systems see themselves as change agents, not just survivors

### *The Radical Emancipation Framework*

The process of Radical Emancipation is not about perfection; it is about the revolution to create change within our connected and imbedded systems through our individual liberation. Couples and intimate relationships will do more than heal; they transform their communities.

## Phase 1: Visioning the Revolution

A guiding question that may support client systems to articulate about the nature of their revolution is, "If your relationship could change the world, what would it change?" This sets the stage for a deep curiosity about the future and possibilities that are present.

Additional questions for exploration:

- "What rules would your love rewrite?"
- "What would children learn from witnessing your partnership?"
- "How does your healing heal your ancestors and support possible descendants?"
- "What becomes possible when you're free?"

## Phase 2: Designing New Realities

Moving from vision to construction offers client systems substantive and concrete methods to view the changes that they have made. Creative options include the following:

1. **Relationship Constitution**: Write your own relationship laws.
2. **Cultural Creation**: Design rituals, celebrations, and traditions.
3. **Community Building**: Gather others in liberation.
4. **Legacy Planning**: How will your freedom outlive you?

### *Clinical Interventions*

The following interventions can be helpful in promoting exercises that help client system embody the work of being and staying free.

## The Freedom Practice

- Morning affirmations of chosen identity. These affirmations can be written, verbal, musically expressive, or artistic in any manner
- Evening celebrations of resistance and upheaval to continue to
- Weekly community gatherings where care can be intertwined ecologically
- Monthly relationship reviews with intimate relationships and family members to highlight the growth and freedom they may have been present
- Annual liberation celebrations

## The LEGO Map

This activity uses LEGOs to build a tangible, 3D representation of the client systems' internal and external worlds. It allows them to physically construct and deconstruct their relationships and sense of impact.

- **The Foundation**: The client begins by building a small, stable structure—perhaps a house or a single figure to represent their **liberated self** as the foundation.
- **The Inner Circle**: They then add smaller LEGO structures or figures immediately around their foundation. Each one can represent a family member(s) or close friend. The client can use different colored bricks to represent the quality of these relationships (e.g., green for expansion, red for challenges).
- **The Community**: The client can then build larger, more complex structures and/or figures further out to represent their **community and friends**. They can use different shapes and sizes to reflect the diversity of these groups (e.g., a "school," a "workplace," a "support group"). They can connect these structures with LEGO roads or bridges to show how they are connected influence wise.
- **The Ripple Effect**: To represent the impact on **strangers and future generations**, the client can create a vast, scattered field of LEGO studs or small, single-brick structures extending from the main map. This visualizes how their positive influence spreads far and wide.

## The Fabric of Connections

This activity uses yarn and a base (e.g., hoop for crocheting) to create a visual web of relationships, symbolizing how the client's healing weaves a new, stronger social tapestry.

- **The Core**: The client starts with a central object, such as a small wooden hoop or a cardboard circle, that represents their **core self**.

- **The Threads**: The client then attaches different colored pieces of yarn to the core object. Each color can represent a different group: a specific color for **family**, another for **friends**, and a third for **community**.
- **The Web**: The client weaves and ties these threads to a larger frame, board, or hoop, creating a web that expands outward. As they talk about the positive influence of their Radical Emancipation, they can use more yarn to connect the different parts of the web, making the pattern more intricate and complex.
- **The Broader Impact**: To represent their influence on **strangers and future generations**, the client can let some of the threads hang loose and extend beyond the main frame or hoop. They can tie small beads or trinkets to these threads to symbolize the "gifts" of love and healing they are sharing with the world.

### *Integration with Community*

Radical Emancipation is a communal action that requires us to connect our freedom back into the communities we exist in. Client systems may do so by:

## Creating Accountability Circles

- Gather other folx in liberation.
- Celebrate rebellions together.
- Hold each other through backlash.

## Becoming Models

- Share story publicly (with safety considerations).
- Mentor others.
- Challenge systems together.
- Create alternative structures.

### *Common Clinical Challenges*

**Challenge**: "This feels too big and/or overwhelming to do."
**MRT Response**: "Revolution happens in daily choices. You do not need to change the entire world, just your world. Start there."
**Challenge**: "We might face real consequences"
**MRT Response**: "Yes that is true. Let's safety plan while we freedom plan. What support do you need? What risks are worth taking? How do we protect your joy?"

## Exercises and Discussion Questions

1 Radical Emancipation is presented as potentially creating "fourth-order change" that transforms communities, not just individuals or relationships. How do you measure and support change that extends beyond your therapy room into clients' broader social networks?
2 This chapter describes Black Queer individuals as creating "realization of relationships grounded in who they were and what they wanted" despite societal rejection. How can you help clients envision and create relationship models that may have no precedent in their experience?
3 Radical Emancipation requires being "free from oppression and interference" to create authentic relationships. How do you help clients identify subtle forms of interference they may not recognize, and what does genuine freedom look like in practice?
4 This chapter notes that this "profound relationship shifting position" builds on all previous MRT interventions. How would you sequence therapeutic work to ensure clients are prepared for the vulnerability and responsibility that Radical Emancipation requires?

# 10 Jamal and Marcus

## MRT with a Queer Couple

### Meeting Jamal and Demarcus

Jamal and Demarcus found me the way many Black Queer couples do—through whispered recommendations in community spaces, through text that said, "after all the searching, we found the one," through the exhausting search for a therapist who wouldn't require them to educate before they could heal. They'd tried therapy twice before. The first therapist, well-meaning but lost, kept asking them to explain basic concepts about gay relationships. The second, a gay white man, couldn't grasp why race mattered in their bedroom dynamics. By the time they sat in my office, Jamal in his company jacket, Demarcus in scrubs from his nursing shift, carried the familiar exhaustion I see in so many Black Queer couples. They are tired of translating lived experiences, tired of code-switching, and tired of being everything to everyone except themselves.

"We love each other," Jamal began, his hand finding Demarcus's across the couch gap, "but something's stuck. We keep having the same fights, and they're getting uglier."

Demarcus nodded, adding, "It's like we're speaking different languages lately. And with everything else we're dealing with…" He trailed off. There was that silence that holds volumes of unspoken hurt and pain.

Their presenting concerns were layered. Each was becoming more complex and intertwined:

- **Surface Level:** Communication breakdowns, sexual dissatisfaction, disagreements about money.
- **Underneath:** Jamal's promotion to the only Black senior engineer at his company had him "performing excellence" to exhaustion.
- **Deeper:** Demarcus's mother had started sending him "pray the gay away" articles after years of tentative acceptance.
- **Core:** They wanted to become fathers but couldn't agree on how—adoption, surrogacy, or remaining child-free.

DOI: 10.4324/9781032725987-10

But underneath all of this lay the fundamental question that brings many Black Queer couples to therapy: How do we love each other fully when the world insists we shouldn't exist?

## Societal Expectations: Unpacking the Luggage

In our third session, we began excavating the societal expectations overcoming their relationship. I pulled out a large paper and drew three circles: one for Jamal, one for Demarcus, and one for their relationship.

"Let's map the expectations," I said. "Not the ones you chose, but the ones forced upon you."

Jamal laughed bitterly. "How much time you got doc?"

We started with workplace expectations. Jamal described his daily code-switching. "I have to be exceptional but not threatening. A strong leader but not too aggressive. I phase in and out of stances so hard that by the time I get home, I don't know which voice is mine anymore."

Demarcus jumped in: "And then he comes home to me expecting him to be this strong, dominant top because that's what Black men are 'supposed' to be, even gay ones. Especially gay ones."

"Whoa," Jamal turned to him. "Is that what you think?"

"Isn't that what you think?" Demarcus shot back.

This moment where the therapist may miss an opportunity to dig deeper into the contextual issues with their client systems is where Multidynamic Relational Therapy (MRT) will shine. The recognition of how societal expectations had infiltrated their most intimate space cracked something open. We spent the rest of the session mapping how anti-Blackness, homophobia, and toxic masculinity had written scripts for their relationship without their consent.

## Values Alignment: Which Way Are They Traveling?

Session six focused on values, but not the surface types, the ones that carry much more weight.

"Beyond what others expect," I asked, "what do you actually value in your love?"

Demarcus went first: "Softness and tenderness. I want us to be soft with each other. The world is so hard on Black men, on Gay men, on Black Gay men. I want our home to be different."

Jamal's eyes welled. "I didn't know you wanted that. I thought… I thought you needed me to be strong all the time."

"When have I ever said that?" Demarcus asked gently.

"You didn't have to. The world said it for you."

We created a values constellation—not a list but a living document of what mattered: Tenderness. Authenticity. Pleasure without performance. Joy as resistance. Family expansion on their own terms.

## Power Analysis: Who Holds What?

The power conversation emerged naturally when discussing their sex life. They'd been stuck in rigid roles based on body types, skin tones, and physical presentations. Jamal was always topping and Demarcus always bottoming. These sexual positions were clearly unexamined assumptions about their bodies.

"Let's map the power," I suggested, pulling out the Power Analysis worksheet.

What we discovered through this intervention:

- Jamal held economic power (higher salary).
- Demarcus held emotional power (more connected to family and community).
- Neither felt they had sexual power (both constrained by stereotypes).
- External power (families, society) dominated internal power.

"What if you could redistribute this?" I asked. "What if power could flow between you rather than be hoarded?"

Demarcus suggested they try switching not just their sexual positions but all their assumed roles. Jamal would plan their social calendar. Demarcus would manage investments. They'd communicate desires without assuming who "should" want what.

## Liberation: Choosing Joy

By session 12, something had shifted. Demarcus came in wearing nail polish—gold and glittering.

"My mom called about it," he said. "Saw it on my story. Said it wasn't godly."

"And?" I prompted.

"And I told her that my God loves all of me, including the parts that sparkle."

Jamal beamed. "Tell him what else you said."

Demarcus grinned. "I said if she couldn't love her gay son with gorgeous nails, that was between her and her God, not me and mine."

This was liberation making itself apparent through choice, not the absence of oppression. Demarcus chose joy over approval. Jamal chose vulnerability over armor. Together, they chose their own definitions over society's limitations.

We processed the grief too as liberation isn't always free. Demarcus mourned the mother he needed but didn't have. Jamal grieved the easier path his straight siblings walked. But in that grief, they found each other more fully.

## Radical Emancipation: Creating What We Want

Session 20 brought us to Radical Emancipation. They'd been doing the work all these weeks challenging expectations, aligning values, sharing power, and choosing liberation. Now came the revolution.

"We want to have a baby," Jamal announced. "But not the way anyone expects."

They'd designed their own path: They would pursue surrogacy, but with Demarcus's sperm first (subverting assumptions about Jamal as the "masculine" one needing biological children). They would raise their child with chosen family as active co-parents. They would teach their child that family is whoever shows up with love and a good meal when you need them.

But bigger than the baby decision was how they'd rewritten their relationship rules:

- Pleasure over performance or productivity in all things.
- Emotions flow freely regardless of who's "supposed" to feel what.
- Their home is a Black Queer sanctuary where code-switching ends at the door.
- Love is their resistance.

## The Transformation

By our final session (number 25), Jamal and Demarcus had become different people, or better said, they showed me freely who they always were without the beratement of society's constraints.

Jamal spoke first: "I cried at work yesterday. In front of my white boss. And you know what? The world didn't end."

Demarcus added: "I topped last night and I loved it. We both did. I might do it again this weekend."

These might seem like small victories, but for Black Gay men navigating multiple oppressive systems, they're revolutionary acts. Every tear Jamal shed chipped away at the stereotype of the dangerous Black man. Every time Demarcus claimed sexual agency, he rewrote scripts about what Black Gay men's bodies are "for."

Their relationship became an exercise to practice freedom. Things were not perfect, but they certainly were free.

## Clinical Reflections

Working with Jamal and Demarcus illuminated MRT's foundational truth. The use of therapeutic models that are attuned to some of the most vulnerable in our community is a powerful tool for healing. Centering Black Queer experiences can do more than help couples in therapy. We can participate in collective liberation. Their healing flowed outward. Jamal started an affinity group for Black engineers at his company. Demarcus began facilitating a support group for Black Gay men with religious trauma. Their future child would grow up knowing that love makes one family, not blood or law or tradition.

This is MRT's promise: Therapy that does more than just heals wounds. It creates conditions to transform worlds.

## Exercises and Discussion Questions

1. How might a therapist's own identity and societal positioning influence their ability to recognize and address the multiple layers of code-switching that Black Queer clients experience? Consider how Jamal's workplace performance of "exceptional but not threatening" masculinity intersected with his relationship dynamics.
2. The case demonstrates how external oppressive systems (racism, homophobia) can rigidly constrain power dynamics within Black Queer relationships, particularly around sexuality and gender expression. How can therapists help client systems move beyond identifying these constraints to actively redistributing power in ways that honor both partners' authentic selves? What are the potential risks and benefits of encouraging clients to experiment with role reversals, and how do you support clients through the vulnerability this requires?
3. Demarcus choosing to wear nail polish despite his mother's disapproval represents "liberation making itself apparent through choice, not the absence of oppression." How does this distinction between liberation and traditional healing models challenge conventional therapeutic outcomes? When working with marginalized clients, how do you balance supporting individual healing with acts of resistance that may increase external conflict but promote authenticity and agency?
4. The case highlights how Jamal and Demarcus grieved "the easier path" and "the mother [Demarcus] needed but didn't have" as part of their liberation process. How can therapists help client systems process the unique grief that comes with choosing forced adaptation over acceptance?
5. Jamal and Demarcus found a therapist who didn't require them to "educate before they could heal." How does the therapeutic relationship itself become a practice ground for the kind of sanctuary these clients seek to create in their homes and communities? What specific modifications to traditional therapeutic approaches might be necessary to ensure that therapy becomes a space where "code-switching ends at the door," and how do these modifications align with or challenge your current clinical training and practice?

# 11 Ballroom

## 10 out of 10

It's a Saturday night in New York City and a party is about the start. Many Queer Black folx and their Muvah and families, known as Houses, will descend upon a space filled with glamorous outfits, makeup done up to the godz and a panel of elders in the community that judge how fabulous these people are. The ball is usually hosted by an master of ceremonies or emcee who often provides commentary for the happenings of each walk and category. Tonight, these Houses must compete in five categories which are themes that govern how the folx will need to dress and what scenes they can use creative interpretations to demonstrate their conceptualization of said theme. The five themes tonight are Face, where the most beautiful face is rewarded. Typically, those who take part in the art of drag or who are trans-female may walk this category. Butch Femme, where individuals must display a masculine appearance within femininity. Studs, lesbian women who……may walk this category. Male Realness. Bizarre, where outfits and concepts of design and interaction are completely outside of what we would consider to be normal and challenge what we may think of as fashion. Lastly there is Legendary, where only the most prominent houses and often the Muvah and/or Father of said Houses are allowed to walk and demonstrate their skill. Often the Legendary Walk is a celebration of said House heads for their position as leaders and caregivers in the community.

When the participants "walk" in the ball, there is a routine that most folx follow. The first is the actual Walk. This walk is not simply strolling down an aisle to get to the audience. It is much more. The slink, the switch, the sensual ways that you demonstrate your sexuality, personhood, and introduction of your interpretation of the category. Think about the presence of actress/model Naomi Campbell on the runway and how you can only see her stage presence. The second portion of the routine is Hands. Participants vogue and move their hands and bodies to continue to tell a story about who they are and what they came to do. Sometimes that handwork is simple and to the point but often it is filled with intricate movements swaying back and forth, behind the back and twirling their arms to match the dynamic emotions that are present. The routine then moves to the Duckwalk which may be one of the most recognizable and mimicked portions. The participant bounces as they walk while crouching

DOI: 10.4324/9781032725987-11

down moving their feet forward, backward, and often jumping up. The culmination of this portion of the routine is usually a Death Drop which is a kick in the air with the person falling to the ground suddenly with one leg tucked and the other extended. This Duckwalk and its portion ender the Death Drop require a great deal of agility, physical awareness, cohesion of your dance, flow with the music being played/MCee'd, and story that you are telling. The audience generally appreciates this portion of the routine and will go wild depending on how fierce a participant(s) is/are. Lastly, the routine moves to the floor where they must demonstrate sensual power and desirability. Many times, there will be head rolling, hair spinning, downward doglike poses that again show off how agile and flexible a person can be. Participants walking the ball in certain categories may walk with someone else in a competition known as a Battle. The two or three people doing their routines must make a demonstration to the judges that they are truly creative in embodying the category above their competitors. The MC, while not a judge, provides a working verbal story and beat for folx to move their bodies to, and even though they are not judges, they may move to Chop a participant if they are only going through the motions, cause confusion and commotion, or simply do not walk a routine that is in that category.

The judges play a critical role in this event. They exist to be wow'd, floored, and impressed. For those that do exceptionally well, judges reward them with tens across the board or ten out of ten. This standard of excellence only comes about for those "who left no crumbs or slayed" all of the competition. The judges also are elders and leaders in the community that kept watchful eyes on the younger generations offering them support, carrying historical knowledge of the LGBTQ+ Black community, giving the Tea (information) of what was going on and creating action plans for support of said community should there be a threat looming (police raids, police targeting).

The happenings of the Ballroom experience are included as an inspiration of the MRT model. Ballroom history is rich and revolutionary and rooted in resistance against oppression of strict white supremacist views on gender, race, sexuality, intimacy, and relationships.

William Dorsey is believed to be the first drag queen in the United States Joseph, C. G. (2021). William was a former slave who began to find individuals like him who wanted to create a safe place for people at that time to do drag shows. Dorsey organized these events and called them Balls. Folx from around the nation and world traveled to participate. Eventually Balls began to pop up in cities like Baltimore and New York City and become exclusionary toward Black and Brown folx because of racism. On top of this, the spaces that were designated as safe spaces began to become targets of police raids as many laws were passed discriminating against Queer people for simply being Queer and gathering. The Black and Brown Queer community began organizing Ballroom events in their own in places such as Harlem which were generally outside of where many of the police raids and law oversight happened

(Bausum, 2016). Because of this, the Black Ballroom movement began to move forward rapidly.

Fast-forward to the 1980s, the AIDS pandemic was in full force, and the United States government turned their backs on the Queer community. Instead of declaring a state of emergency, Queer people who became HIV (then known just as AIDS) positive and fell sick were ostracized by their families and narratives about God's judgment rained supreme. Other narratives were that this was a fearful time for everyone as the understanding about HIV and its transmission were poorly understood. The Queer community knew that it had to survive and to do that began to take care of themselves and those who had lost connections with their biological counterparts who would have potentially came forward to support those who were dying and/or needed support. While the federal and state governments eventually formulated a response and began to instill support to both track and create funding for research, support, and medication, it was only after the Queer community stepped in to support their own (Piot, 2006).

The Black Queer community began to organize themselves into what are called Houses. These Houses were groups of folx who competed together in balls, but they were also chosen family. They were a group of folx who banded together based on similar interests, life narratives, or even appreciations of certain forms of fashion to support each other emotionally and financially. They knew that the power of a chosen community could overcome anything. The heads of these Houses were called Mothers (Muvahs) and Fathers (Favas). These parental figures were leaders in the Queer community and could provide maternal and parental support to the younger Queer folx who were navigating circumstances of ostracization from their biological homes and families, understanding and embracing their sexual and gender identities while figuring out how to make sense of the atrocity in losing friends and other families members to the AIDS epidemic.

MRT pulls on the rich history and traditions of Ballroom culture. To compete in Ballroom, to exist in Ballroom, and to organize houses in Ballroom were all acts of revolution and defiance against the incredible push from those in power who dared to define human expression not from a place of divinity or love but from the position of another human person who often dehumanized other humans. The tenets and assumptions within MRT align themselves with the language and pathway that Black Queer folx have paved as a roadmap for happiness, satisfaction, and victory in relationships and communities.

Ballroom culture inspires MRT as it models how marginalized communities create liberation through collective creativity. The Houses that saved Black Queer youth during the AIDS crisis demonstrate MRT's core principle: community care in the face of social adversity that is rooted in dehumanization will always be the preferred way forward. When biological families failed, they created chosen families. When society denied then their humanity, they defied the odds and validated their identities.

Every element of Ballroom appears in MRT's clinical application. Whoever walks the ball in what category they desire is actively flipping Societal Expectations on their head. A cisgender heterosexual man can like pink and bop out to the "feminine" song on the charts, express his emotions in healthy ways, and be secure in his sexuality. For this heterosexual man to "walk the categories" he wants and find joy in the expression of himself regardless of what the social script for a heterosexual male is to see Ballroom's Values Alignment play out in motion. The Houses model Power Analysis and Sharing—Mothers and Fathers holding power not to dominate but to nurture, protect, and launch the next generation. Liberation happens every time someone walks their truth down that runway. And Radical Emancipation? That's the moment a person realizes that the community they have built through the authentic expression of self brings about true joy in their lives.

MRT brings Ballroom's wisdom into the therapy room. We help individuals, intimate relationships, and families become their own Houses, write their own categories, and choose their own expression of love that works for them. Every Black Queer couple that achieves their own tens across the board proves what Ballroom has always known: excellence isn't about society's must-do's but transcending them entirely.

**Exercises and Discussion Questions**

1 Ballroom culture is presented as inspirational for MRT due to its roots in "resistance against oppression." How can you incorporate the celebratory, affirming aspects of Ballroom culture into your therapeutic practice while respecting the cultural origins?
2 The concept of "Houses" as chosen family providing "maternal and parental support" offers an alternative to traditional family structures. How do you help clients create and maintain chosen family systems when biological families are unsupportive or harmful?
3 Ballroom performance requires "agility, physical awareness, cohesion of dance, flow with music, and storytelling." How might these same skills translate to relationship building and therapeutic work?
4 Ballroom emerged as a response to exclusion from white-dominated spaces and police targeting. How do current therapeutic institutions potentially replicate these exclusionary practices, and what would inclusive, culturally affirming therapy spaces look like?

# 12 MRT and Family Therapy

## From Individuals to Relationships

The field of psychotherapy and adjacent fields have experienced an evolution over the last 100 years. Not so long ago, much of therapy focused solely on the individual—diving deep into their subconscious, their past experiences, and their personal struggles. Psychotherapy contained interventions where the spotlight was almost entirely on the client as a solitary entity. While incredibly valuable, Psychoanalytic approaches often are ill-equipped to tackle the messy and interconnected realities of human relationships.

Then came a powerful shift. We began to incorporate an already existing philosophy and acknowledgment that people don't exist in a vacuum. Our experiences, our struggles, and our well-being are shaped by our relationships and the larger systems we're part of. This realization was largely sparked by ideas like General Systems Theory (GST) and cybernetics – terminology that transcends the therapy space and generally defines that everything is connected.

This new way of thinking birthed Systemic Family Therapy (SFT), which transformed how individuals, intimate relationships, and families received treatment. It offered therapists the opportunity to examine not only the individual issues that may have contributed to their problem but also the communication patterns, unspoken rules, relational responses, and the interconnected and complex ways that acceptance and rejection appear in relationships.

Enter Multidynamic Relational Therapy (MRT). This model was created to create an inclusive model of therapy that truly grounds and supports Queer relationships. While many therapeutic models attempt to be inclusive by reverse engineering their framework that is based in heteronormative standards and representing their models work clinical research, MRT begins by centering Queer identities, unique dynamics, people of color, and diverse relationship structures. In this chapter, you will see how MRT isn't just "inclusive"; it is truly a companion to systemic sex therapy. You will also examine key ideas and interventions, showing you how MRT can be a powerful theory in your practice of therapy working with all kinds of relationships, especially those in the Queer community.

DOI: 10.4324/9781032725987-12

## The Core Ideas That Shape MRT

Before we dive into the use of MRT as an SFT model, a review of the fundamental tenets and terminology of systemic thinking may be helpful to understand the theoretical world of systemic intervention.

At its heart, systemic therapy rests on GST (Skyttner, 1996). Our biological bodies are a great example of understanding GST. The numerous parts of our human bodies carry out various tasks and functions; however, none of them operate in isolation. Each part (heart, brain, stomach, intestine, etc.) is interconnected to another and often operates in tandem with other parts to create an intricate system. GST argues that our world is holistic and made up of sophisticated systems. When this is applied to the human experience, the individual contains their own function, but they are influenced by others in their community and vice versa. If change were to occur in one part of the system, it would impact everything else connected to it. "The whole is other than the sum of its parts" (Koffka, 2013).

Maintaining a systemic lens in the practice of therapy is crucial. Consider the conversations that appear with individual clients, couples, and other intimate relational structures as well as families. We limit our understanding of their struggles in strengths as the focus may be linear. SFT helps us avoid that trap by expanding our understanding of the system that the client is within. From there we have more pathways to support the client. It pushes us beyond simply breaking problems down into individual pieces. Invites us to see the intricate dance of interactions, the way people communicate (and don't communicate!), and the shared purpose that keeps the system going.

Every system, regardless of who is in the room with a therapist, has three key features:

1 **The Players (Elements)**: These are the individual people in the system—the family members and the partners.
2 **The Connections (Interconnections)**: They relate to each other through these connections. Communication is passed via these pathways. These are also the dynamic (rules and roles) that bind them in the system.
3 **The Underlying Goal (Shared Purpose)**: This is the unspoken (or sometimes explicit) reason the system operates in the manner it does. Many times, meaning making has been made in order to create this shared purpose. These purposes can be healthy, unhealthy, or a combination of both.

Systemic therapists do not intervene to "fix" the individual but support the entirety of the system to shift. Why is this the case? Often first-order change, or individual behavioral-based change, will only go so far and will not always sustain. This change is also complicated as the system the individual is bound to will always revert to their baseline or homeostasis. However, should the system be supported in changing, individual changes, be it behavioral or relational, have a greater chance of lasting.

One other vital concept in systemic work is the difference between "content" and "process." During sessions, the client system generally brings us "content"—the specific details of what they're discussing (e.g., "We fought about who does the dishes," or "My boss gave me a bad review."). But as systemic therapists, we're listening for and to the "process," meaning how the dynamics that enforce the issues they may be facing. This can include body language, tone of voice, who interrupts whom, who avoids contributing to conversations and when they might, and the underlying relational dynamics at play. This "how" is often called "metacommunication"—it's the communication about the communication itself (Hass-Cohen et al., 2017). We pay close attention to these process-level interactions because they often reveal the deeper patterns and unspoken rules that govern the system, far more than the actual topic of conversation. For instance, a couple arguing about money might actually be enacting a deeper struggle for control or an avoidance of intimacy.

## MRT: An SFT Model

MRT emerged from a clear need to create a model of therapy that centers Queer people of color. This model is appropriate for intimate relationships but also for families. MRT's five tenets function within systemic knowledge and intervention and naturally can be used to support families who are attempting to change and tackle problems but are having trouble with how to shift into a more flexible and healthy dynamic.

The sections below will provide an example of how to utilize this model via the five tenets with families as a systemic model. MRT flows like water in a stream; it flows differently with each family it touches, honoring their unique rhythm and customs. The model is respectful of the family culture and will enrich the customs inherent in the system that create a sense of belonging and shared identity.

## Systemic Application of MRT with Families

Each of MRT's five tenets gives us a specific way to understand and intervene in the relational system, offering actionable pathways for therapists:

1 **Societal Expectations**: MRT recognizes that the world outside our clients' doors profoundly shapes their relationships. Societal expectations dictate roles, dynamics, and even unspoken rules within partnerships. Consider the sway of heteronormative or cisnormativity ideas subtly (or not so subtly) influencing everything from who will engage in the emotional labor of the relationship or the duties one may carry based on their perceived gender or their sex. These expectations often carry the weight of family

history and cultural norms, creating pressures that can lead to unhealthy patterns and conflict if not openly discussed and collaboratively agreed upon.

From a systemic viewpoint, Societal Expectations are powerful external systems constantly interacting with and impacting the internal workings of a family system. An MRT therapist will support them in identifying these external pressures, exploring their origins, and consciously choosing how they want to define their own roles, rather than unconsciously following harmful scripts that may not align to how they desire their family to function. Families will be empowered to create a relational family unit that truly reflects *them*, not society's blueprint.

2 **Values Alignment**: MRT emphasizes that for any intimate relationship to truly thrive, families need to be on the same page about their core values. Values are the moral and ethical compass that guides a relational system—they influence decisions about connection, the right to develop in a specific manner, spirituality, identity, and how they spend their time. In a systemic sense, shared values contribute to the "purpose" that holds a relationship together. When values clash and lack consent or when family members assume shared values are held by everyone in the system, it can create friction or be seen behaviorally as disobedience or obstinance. This will often show up as recurring arguments, power struggles, and a feeling of being stuck with both parents and children.

MRT provides therapists the opportunity to uncover, articulate, and negotiate these core values within the family system. It gives them permission to be real about what matters by naming it and figuring out how everyone in the family can honor what is important to each other. This means going beyond surface-level topics like compliance to explore what may matter to each person. This process fosters a stronger sense of shared purpose and cohesion within the family system. For example, parents may have a vision and mindset of how their child(ren) should engage with the school system when entering High School. Parents may expect their children to join several clubs, stay busy with sports and other activities, make friends, find a job, do well in classes, be ready for college, and at least ponder on what sort of major they would want in college. Without discussing this openly and soliciting consent from their children regarding this plan, their differing values could lead to constant tension over the child's trajectory in school. A therapist utilizing this model would facilitate a dialogue to create an opportunity for the family to discuss these underlying values, validate existing perspectives, and then collaboratively create a shared understanding that honors both the values of all parties. This strengthens the overall cohesion of their relationship.

3 **Power Analysis**: MRT asserts a fundamental truth: power exists in all relationships, whether we acknowledge it or not. For relationships to be truly healthy and equitable, power needs to be consciously shared and openly

discussed between partners. Systemically, power dynamics are woven into the threads and fabric of how families connect and interact. Power isn't just about control; it's about who influences decisions, whose needs get prioritized, how disagreements are settled, and whose reality is validated. When there is a power imbalance, especially those that are unexamined, it leads to rigid patterns, communication breakdowns, resentment, and overall dysfunction in the family system. These imbalances can come from societal norms (like traditional gender roles or economic differences), individual personalities, or even long-standing patterns that are passed down intergenerationally.

MRT's Power Analysis encourages families to explicitly identify and negotiate how power plays out in the family system and interpersonal relationships. This involves asking questions like: How do you as parents involve the family in making system altering decisions? Whose voice(s) carries more weight? How do we resolve conflicts and encourage repair between individuals? How can I as a parent help embody consensual decision-making in relationships? By bringing these implicit power structures to the therapy room and acknowledging them as a process to engage in, MRT helps families create a more balanced and respectful distribution of power. Now, not every family believes that power should be shared. Some families carry traditions, some carry trauma, and some carry both. Therapists are still free to utilize this with families and gain consent from those who hold power on how the distribution and sharing of power can take shape.

4 **Liberation**: MRT defines Liberation as a profound journey where individuals actively challenge harmful and limiting societal expectations and take ownership of their sense of self and determination within the family relationship. This systemic concept is intertwined with the previous tenets. Family members can confront how issues such as internalized homophobia, transphobia, racism, sexism, or other forms of marginalization act as an invisible (and many times visible) force and barrier that distort and limits familial relationships. These oppressive patterns if left unchecked can often create rigid, unhealthy "rules" or "purposes" with families, stifling authenticity, agency, growth, and the ability to create healthy interactions and expectations.

Liberation, then, is an active process of creating and sustaining space to be free. It is the dismantling of internalized narratives, self-limiting beliefs, and the external pressures imposed by oppressive societal structure. It means reclaiming agency, time, and prioritizing embrace ways that are true to oneself, rather than conforming to damaging external scripts. When members in a system allow for liberation to set place within their family system, this produces intent for the system to welcome each person to contribute to the shared purpose from a place of authenticity. This acceptance allows for full participation in the family system that creates a safe place for individuals to exercise freedom.

5 **Radical Emancipation**: As the final and most expansive tenet, Radical Emancipation represents the ultimate transformation: a complete revision and re-creation of one's relationships, their rules, and their roles. This stems directly from the deep work done in the liberation process. This step when used as a systemic model with families creates movement toward **fourth-order** change. That is to say, the family has found a new way of relating and identifying a way to exist, thrive, and find happiness and harmony within the family system despite the larger societal and global challenges.

Radical Emancipation is the systemic goal of the successful use of MRT. It signifies a state where individuals and their relationships have fundamentally restructured and redefined themselves, truly free from the constraints of harmful societal expectations and oppressive dynamics. Solving problems is not the focus of this step; it's about *consciously co-creating* a new relational reality. It involves deliberately establishing new ways of relating, crafting new relational rules that reflect their wishes for interdependent relationships within the family, and consistently magnifying a new, self-determined shared purpose that prioritizes authenticity, equity, and mutual liberation for all participants.

## Incorporating MRT in Your Therapy

MRT's core philosophy is clear: problems in any of its five areas—Societal Expectations, Values, Power Analysis, Liberation, or Radical Emancipation—don't exist in isolation. There is overlap and it will create conflict and limits within relationships. This interconnectedness is a hallmark of systemic philosophy and intervention. Symptoms and their influence not only impact a person of the individual level but ripple within the family, intimate, and greater system of that individual.

Here are a few ways you can incorporate MRT within your systemic work:

- **Identify the Greater Story and Dynamic (Process over Content)**: While clients will bring you the "content" of their issues (e.g., "We always fight about money," or "They never listen to me"), an MRT therapist will not only listen and look for the "process" by asking questions such as: *How* do they fight about money? *How* do they interrupt each other? *What* is the underlying dynamic when one person feels unheard? They will also explore the influence of societal expectations, misaligned values, or unspoken power dynamics. MRT shifts the focus from a tit-for-tat argument to the deeper, underlying interactive processes that fuel divergence in relationships.

- **Reframing Symptoms, Systemically**: MRT offers a powerful way to reframe relational "symptoms." Instead of seeing a child's withdrawal as disrespect or disregard for family norms, an MRT therapist might reframe it as a systemic response to an unacknowledged power imbalance, or a reaction to an ingrained societal expectation about how emotions should be expressed. This crucial reframing shifts the "blame" from an individual to the entire relational system and its broader influences.
- **Intervening on Multiple Levels**: As systemic therapists, we know that the most impactful changes happen when we support relationships and the entirety of a system, not just the individuals. MRT excels here. It validates individual experiences and the use of it as the primary theoretical framework can provide a healthy shift in fundamental interconnections (through addressing Societal Expectations, Values, and Power Analysis). Moreover, it aims to change the very purpose and rules of the relationship through Liberation and Radical Emancipation. The ability for a therapist to offer this as an outcome creates greater healing for those you treat.
- **Relationships, Even in Individual Work**: Even when you're working with an individual client, MRT encourages you to keep a relational lens. You'd explore how their personal struggles are shaped by their past and present relationships, societal "norms" and pressure, and internalized relational dynamics via their family of origin. The goal is not only to promote wellness within the individual, but facilitating systemic shifts in how they understand themselves *within their relational world*, empowering them to change their interactions and responses.

## Conclusion: MRT's Vital Role in Modern Systemic Therapy

MRT is more than just another therapy model; it's a vital, timely, and unique addition to our systemic toolkit, especially because of its intentional and explicit focus on the dynamic that resides within Queer relationships. By integrating the core principles of GST and skillfully using systemic techniques, MRT gives us a comprehensive, flexible, and culturally attuned framework for understanding and effectively intervening in the often-complex dynamics of family work.

Its five foundational interventions—Societal Expectations, Values, Power Analysis, Liberation, and Radical Emancipation—are more than abstract concepts or theoretical tenets; they are practical entry points into the heart of a relationship's systemic workings. Together, these tenets help us address the intricate dance between individuals, the nuanced structures of their family dynamics, and the broader societal and cultural forces that constantly shape them. MRT goes beyond the application of systemic principles; it embodies them, recognizing that relational struggles are never isolated, but rather emerge from and are maintained by complex systemic interactions.

Most importantly, MRT offers a clear, structured, and deeply empowering path toward profound transformation for humans, given the timeline that we are experiencing right now, the ability to fundamentally change their relationships with themselves, their families and the greater communities they reside in. It provides a clear pathway for larger political, complex, and sometimes oppressive topics to not be seen as a side conversation in therapy, but one that can be readily grappled with in the course of our fifty (50) minute sessions.

As the field of psychotherapy as well as systemic therapy continues to grow and embrace the incredible diversity of human experience, MRT stands out as a powerful, attuned, and essential theoretical framework to foster health, equity, and freedom for all human relationships. Its development marks a significant step forward in ensuring that therapeutic models are truly inclusive, effective, and capable of addressing the full spectrum of relational complexities we encounter in our practice.

## Exercises and Discussion Questions

1 MRT "flows like water in a stream, flowing differently with each family it touches." How do you balance this fluid, adaptive approach with the need for clinical structure and measurable outcomes in family therapy? What specific assessment tools would help you determine which MRT tenet to prioritize with different family systems?
2 This chapter presents Power Analysis in families as including children's voices in "system altering decisions." How do you implement this practically while maintaining appropriate parental authority? What does "consensual decision-making" look like across different developmental stages and family structures?
3 When working with families where some members hold traditional religious or cultural values that conflict with MRT's liberation principles, how do you honor family values while still addressing internalized oppression? What's your role when parents' beliefs may be limiting their LGBTQ+ child's authenticity?
4 MRT emphasizes that symptoms are systemic responses rather than individual problems. Using a current family case, how would you reframe a presenting problem (like a teen's "acting out") through each of the five MRT tenets? How does this reframing change your intervention strategies?

# 13 MRT in Intimate Relationships and Sex Therapy

Sex therapists stand at a fascinating point in the evolution of our specialized practice. For a time, the focus of sex therapy laid primarily on the individual and that individual's problem. We delved into personal histories, explored inner conflicts, and their medical interventions and background as isolated beings. This approach, while foundational, is incomplete when confronted with the intricate, interconnected realities of human sexuality. What started with a focus on individual physiological responses and behavioral techniques has increasingly evolved into the vast relational, psychological, and societal layers that shape our sexual identities. Despite this much needed growth, there remained still a significant gap, particularly when it comes to intervening and affirming the diverse sexual experiences and sexual wellness of Queer, Black, People of Color as individuals and their relationships via a theoretical model.

Multidynamic Relational Therapy (MRT) was crafted to meet this need. It was specifically created to address this gap, offering a model that centers Queer identities, dynamics, and relationship structures. In this chapter, we'll explore the landscape of sex therapy, discover what makes a sex therapy approach systemic, and why MRT is an essential companion framework for any therapist addressing issues related to sexuality as a sex therapist or not.

## What Is Sex Therapy? An Overview for the Practitioner

In its essence, sex therapy is a specialized form of psychotherapy that assists individuals and relational units of all constellations address concerns related to sexual function, desire, intimacy, and sexual expression (Hertlein et al., 2009). This specialization has grown exponentially since its inception, transcending a purely medical/behavioral focus to embrace a more holistic, biopsychosocial understanding of sexuality.

Historically, sex therapy gained significant traction with the work completed by Masters and Johnson in the 1960s and 1970s. Their innovative and insightful research on the human sexual response cycle was and is the blueprint for many behavioral interventions (Masters & Johnson, 1966). The Masters and Johnson approach, while revolutionary for its time, primarily focused

DOI: 10.4324/9781032725987-13

on treating sexual "dysfunctions" through direct behavioral interventions, often with the "asymptomatic" partner acting as a co-therapist (Masters & Johnson, 1970). While this approach provided success for many couples, this approach was often criticized for multiple reasons with a chief complaint that treated the individual problem rather than the relational context. Helen Singer Kaplan later attempted to bridge the gap between psychodynamic and behavioral approaches, acknowledging relational conflict but sometimes using a "bypass" technique to focus on individual sexual symptoms (Kaplan & Klein, 2014).

Today, the practice of sex therapy is far more nuanced. Many of the trainings and sex therapy theory classes recognize that sexual issues are not solely about the mechanics or the physical body; they are entwined with our thoughts, feelings, relationships, family of origin, and community/societal influences. The specialization has largely adopted a biopsychosocial model, which means considering (Lynn et al., 2023; Nimbi et al., 2022; McCarthy & Wald, 2017):

**Biological Factors**: These include hormonal imbalances, medical conditions, medication side effects, or physical pain that might impact sexual function or desire.

**Psychological Factors**: These include anxiety, depression, trauma (both "large-T" and "small-t" traumas, like infidelity, which can profoundly impact trust and intimacy), body image issues, past sexual experiences, sexual scripts, and individual beliefs about sex.

**Social/Relational Factors**: These encompass communication patterns, relationship dynamics, cultural norms, religious beliefs, family-of-origin messages about sex, and societal expectations around gender and sexuality.

### *Types of Issues Treated in Sex Therapy*

Within the use of the biopsychosocial model of assessment and treatment, sex therapists work with a wide array of concerns, including but not limited to (Tripodi et al., 2022):

- **Desire Discrepancy**: When partners have different levels of sexual interest.
- **Low/Absent Sexual Desire**: Often referred to as Hypoactive Sexual Desire Disorder (HSDD) or Female Sexual Interest/Arousal Disorder (FSIAD).
- **Erectile Dysfunction (ED)**: Difficulty achieving or maintaining an erection.
- **Premature Ejaculation (PE)**: Ejaculating sooner than desired.
- **Orgasmic Difficulties**: Anorgasmia (difficulty reaching orgasm) in any gender.

- **Painful Sex (Dyspareunia/Vaginismus)**: Pain during intercourse or involuntary muscle spasms that prevent penetration.
- **Communication Issues around Sex**: Difficulty discussing sexual needs, desires, or boundaries.
- **Sexual Trauma**: Healing from past sexual abuse, assault, or other traumatic sexual experiences.
- **Infidelity**: Navigating the aftermath of betrayal, which can often be a traumatic attachment injury for both partners.
- **Sexual Identity and Orientation Concerns**: Exploring one's sexual identity, coming out, or navigating relationships that fall outside traditional norms.
- **Body Image Concerns**: How self-perception impacts sexual confidence and pleasure.
- **Out of Control Sexual Behavior**: Patterns of sexual behavior that feel out of control.
- **Impact of Illness or Disability on Sexuality**: Adapting sexual life to chronic health conditions.
- **Exploring Sexual Pleasure and Satisfaction**: Moving beyond dysfunction to enhance positive sexual experiences.

### *Common Modalities and Techniques in Sex Therapy*

Most practice of sex therapy currently is integrative, drawing from various therapeutic approaches to meet the unique needs of relational client systems. The richness of each of the existing models and approaches has in various ways pushed the boundaries to expand into relational work in sex therapy. Some common modalities and techniques include:

**Sensate Focus**: Originally developed by Masters and Johnson, this is a cornerstone technique. It involves structured touch exercises, often starting with nongenital touch, to reduce performance anxiety, increase body awareness, and improve communication about pleasure. It's about focusing on sensation rather than outcome. Modern adaptations often incorporate mindfulness and emphasize mutual enjoyment between the participants (Weiner & Avery-Clark, 2014).

**Cognitive-Behavioral Therapy (CBT)**: Addressing negative thoughts, and assumptions about sex, the self and beliefs of what others may think about them that contribute to sexual difficulties. This might involve challenging irrational fears or reframing self-criticism (Berry, 2013).

**Psychoeducation**: Providing accurate information about sexual anatomy, physiology, common sexual responses, and dispelling myths. This intervention can be an affirmative and normalizing experience for clients (Tahan et al., 2020).

**Mindfulness**: Encouraging present-moment awareness during sexual activity to reduce distraction, reduce performance anxiety, and enhance pleasure (Mize, 2015).

**Communication Skills Training**: Teaching partners how to express their desires, boundaries, and concerns effectively and empathetically. Imago therapy is one of the most recognized models within these techniques (Everaerd & Dekker, 1981).

**Narrative Therapy**: Helping client systems "externalize" the sexual problem (seeing it as separate from themselves) and "re-author" their sexual stories, focusing on unique outcomes and preferred narratives of their sexual selves (Muruthi et al., 2018).

**Emotionally Focused Therapy (EFT)**: For couples, EFT helps identify and transform negative interactional cycles driven by attachment fears, fostering deeper emotional connection and security, which often improves sexual intimacy (Johnson & Zuccarini, 2011).

**Eye Movement Desensitization and Reprocessing (EMDR)**: Increasingly used to process sexual trauma, infidelity-related traumas, or painful experiences that impact sexual health. EMDR helps clients reprocess distressing memories, reducing their emotional charge (Baird, 2021).

**Integrative Approaches**: Many sex therapists identify as integrative, artfully blending techniques from various models and frameworks to offer specified and customized treatment to the client system. There is a growing trend that therapists are more integrative in their practice. A clinical study in 2015 identified that many psychotherapists utilize more than one model or theory in their work (Zarbo et al., 2016; Weeks, 2005).

## Systemic Sex Therapy—It's about You AND Me

The idea of "systemic sex therapy" is a fundamental shift in how we understand and approach sexual concerns and sexual wellness. As stated previously, traditional sex therapy often focused on individual symptoms and intervention occurs in one dimension. Systemic sex therapy conceptualizes sexual issues as inextricably linked to the broader relational and contextual systems in which they occur. It moves beyond the idea that a sexual problem resides solely within one person and offers therapists the ability to investigate and support any relational dynamics that may contribute to symptomology.

The Intersystem Approach is a prime example of a systemic theoretical model that has made significant inroads in bridging the lack of systemic intervention within the traditional sex therapy. It accentuates the integration of sex and couple therapy, arguing that sexual and relational satisfactions are mutually significant. This approach highlights five key domains that intermingle to shape human behavior and relationships, including sexuality (Weeks et al., 2019):

1 **Individual-Biological/Medical**: Recognizing the physical health and biological makeup of each partner.
2 **Individual-Psychological:** Exploring each partner's unique personality, beliefs, attitudes, and psychological history.
3 **Dyadic Relationship/Couple Dynamics**: Exploratory assessment on how partners interact, communicate, manage conflict, and experience intimacy.

This is where the "couple as a system" is elevated as and validated as the unit receiving treatment.

4 **Intergenerational Influences (Family-of-Origin)**: Becoming knowledgeable of how messages, patterns, and values about relationships and sexuality are passed down through generations.
5 **Contextual Factors**: Recognizing the prevailing impact of broader societal, cultural, historical, and religious and spiritual influences, as well as the immediate physical environment.

An advantage of a systemic approach to sex therapy like the Intersystem Approach is its holistic view on treatment of the relational unit. It recognizes that a lack of sexual desire in one partner may indeed be biological issues, but it may also extend to or originate from unresolved relationship conflict, family-of-origin narratives about one's sexuality or the function of sex or societal expectations around sexual performance. The use of a systemic model within the practice of sex therapy offers a wide-ranging of options for the clinician and multiple pathways toward healing and wellness via equifinality.

Despite the growing recognition and application of systemic knowledge within therapeutic models and practitioners, there have been historical challenges in fully integrating the treatment of sexual issues and couple therapy (Lebow & Snyder, 2022). Training programs diverge in what models and philosophies they choose to teach within their classes, professional organizations have operated in insolation and silos, and the actual practice of sex and couple therapy differs in real-life conditions leading to applications that lack fidelity. This lack of comprehensive training can lead to inconsistent care with client systems where clinicians do not have the proper support at bridging the research to practice divide.

## MRT—A Powerful Companion to Systemic Sex Therapy

MRT is a model that not only incorporates systemic principles but advances the boundaries of how systemic sex therapy is applied, particularly for Queer individuals and their relationships. MRT was born from a critical observation; many existing therapeutic models were not created with Queer or People of Color in mind. This can be seen in part where many of the tenets of these models are heteronormative in nature and the advent of clinical research where outcomes studies of models highlight that Queer and/or couples of color found similar positive outcomes in therapy as their heterosexual counterparts. While it is helpful to demonstrate what may be successful for communities in therapy, this has left Queer and People of Color and their relationships feeling unseen and forced to adapt their experiences to a heteronormative framework.

MRT steps into this space, offering a systemic approach native to the relationships of Queer Black relationships. The five tenets and theoretical assumptions provide the sex therapist the ability to understand and intervene in the complexities of human sexuality while centering contextual issues (such as intersecting identities of race, ethnicity, culture, sexual identity, sexual orientation, and neurodiversity) of the client and support the effective use of the therapist's experience as a tool in the treatment of the client system.

Below we will examine of how each of the tenets of MRT can be used as an essential clinical model for systemic sex therapy.

### *Societal Expectations*

MRT allows therapists to observe and name how societal expectations profoundly shape our relationships, including our sexual lives. These expectations often carry the weight of family history, cultural norms, and pervasive biases like heteronormativity and cisnormativity. In sex therapy, this means recognizing how external pressures can dictate "normal" sexual behavior, how gender roles in intimacy take hold, or even how desire "should" manifest. For Queer individuals, these expectations can be particularly sinister, leading to internalized shame, performance anxiety, or a feeling that their natural desires are "wrong."

An MRT-informed sex therapist applying the societal expectations intervention with a potential issue around low desire would branch past the initial complaint. They would explore larger societal narratives and forces that dictate what is considered good sex, who should initiate, or what the physical makeup of dom top looks like and how it may interfere with their levels of desire. This intervention may also involve peeling back those tired heteronormative scripts about roles that say who should want what, who should ask for what, who should give, and who should receive. These scripts are often written for someone else's ideal of sexual intimacy. MRT empowers clients, as well as therapists, to identify these external burdens, challenge their influence, and consciously create their own sexual narratives and practices, free from the constraints of societal pressures that limit expression. This is vital for fostering congruence in sexual intimacy and pleasure.

### *Values Alignment*

MRT underscores that healthy intimate and sexual relationships require a consensual alignment of values between partners. In sex therapy, this would surpass having basic conversations about sexual acts and incorporate what each partner may *believe* is essential in their connection which may motivate the sexual expression of said act. Questions such as: What does "intimacy" mean to each person? What are the core values around matters such as trust, vulnerability, commitment, pleasure, and exploration? When these values are misaligned, assumed, or left acknowledged, they can create conflict in sexual connections which may cascade into unmet needs and experience dissatisfaction in the relationship.

An MRT sex therapist simplifies a complex and nuanced conversation to create an avenue for partners to clarify their values. For example, one partner may place importance in being sexually adventurous and experiencing new sensations, while the other or others give precedence to emotional security and routine. Without conscious alignment, these differences will lead to sexual frustration or unfulfillment. MRT helps the intimate relational constellation convey their personal sexual values, validate each other's perspectives, and then collaboratively build a shared ethos that honors all individuals. This process strengthens the faith each partner has in the sexual system by building a foundation of mutual understanding and respect, allowing for a more fulfilling and congruent sexual life.

### *Power Analysis*

MRT asserts that power dynamics are ever-present in relationships, including sexual ones, and that healthy relationships require a clear and accessible protocol of how to share power. In sex therapy, this is a critical lens. Power lives within many of the sexual issues that are present in therapy. Who initiates sex? Who sets the boundaries of certain activities and why? Whose pleasure is prioritized? Who feels more comfortable expressing desires or saying "no"? Imbalances of power within sexual relationships can manifest as sexual dysfunction, resentment, or a lack of agency for partners. These imbalances can often be exasperated as they are influenced by societal expectations (e.g., gender-related sexual roles, race/ethnicity, and sexual desire) or sexual scripts and narratives that have been passed down by family of origin.

The use of the Power Analysis within MRT in sex therapy allows therapist to openly discuss who holds what kind of power, how it's expressed, and its impact on their sexual interactions. Issues such as initiating sexual experiences can be unpacked in a direct and supportive manner that would allow the client system to engage in a negotiation of sexual interactions with equity. It would also support proper conversation around moving from power-over to power-with which aids the client system in reproducing positive outcomes of future sexual issues.

### *Liberation*

MRT defines Liberation as the process of actively challenging oppression and reforming one's relationship with it. Its use within sex therapy supports recognizing how internalized homophobia, transphobia, racism, sexism, or other forms of oppression modifies a person's sense of their sexual self and their sexual experiences. Oppressive societal messages create shame, anxiety, and a sense of being "broken" sexually, leading to dysfunction or avoidance.

Liberation via MRT in sex therapy is about empowering clients to purge these oppressive narratives in their sexual script. Liberation allows clients to reclaim their sexual agency and pleasure, defining their relationship structure based on their own desires despite the oppression focused on them. An MRT sex therapist helps clients identify how these larger systemic forces are unveiled in their sexual lives and supports them to resist them by creating internalized happiness within.

### *Radical Emancipation*

As the peak of the MRT process, Radical Emancipation represents a profound, fourth-order change in a relationship's sexual landscape. It is about rewriting and re-creating the relationship's sexual rules, roles, and narratives, born from the work completed within the Liberation intervention. This step elevates treatment beyond the abatement of sexual symptoms and dysfunction and allows for a large degree of sexual freedom.

In the practice of sex therapy, Radical Emancipation supports client systems to address the "tolerable sex" (Schnarch, 1991) they may be having and actively craft sexual relationships that are vibrant, satisfying, and imbued with consensual agency. It creates permission for the sexual script to be fluid, exploratory, and connected to shared values and desires, liberated from external pressures. It's about designing a sexual system that is their own, leading to a sense of sexual wellness and pleasure.

## Why MRT Is Essential for Modern Sex Therapy

The field of psychotherapy has increasingly embraced integration, moving away from the rigid adherence to single theories. As John C. Norcross highlights, the sheer "proliferation of therapies" and the "inadequacy of single theories" have driven therapists to look across theoretical boundaries (Norcross & Alexander, 2005). The argument here is not a defense for therapists to be atheoretical in the practice of therapy or sex therapy. It is about acknowledging that our therapeutic models and the variety of our toolbox should be diverse and inclusive. The goal of expanding the options therapists have to treat the ever-diversifying population is to ensure that our clients have a clear reflection of themselves and their lives within the available models.

MRT embodies this integrative spirit, offering a robust framework that innately lends itself to a comprehensive practice of sex therapy. Below are a few additional points that justify the integration of MRT into the practice of sex therapy.

**Addresses Systemic Roots of Sexual Issues**: MRT's core tenets ensure that sexual problems are never viewed in isolation from external circumstances. It requires therapists to explore how societal expectations, power dynamics, and family-of-origin issues directly impact sexual desire, function, and satisfaction. This systemic lens provides a more comprehensive understanding, leading to more sustainable change than an individual or behavioral-based approach.

**Culturally Attunement**: A significant strength of MRT is its explicit centering of Queer and Black identities and experiences. It acknowledges that traditional models fail to capture the unique tribulations and resilience factors for Queer people of color who navigate compounding systems of oppression (racism, heterosexism, cisnormativity, transphobia). MRT provides a framework to address these oppressions directly, making justice and resilience central to sexual wellness.

**Beyond Dysfunction to Pleasure and Wellness**: Many traditional sex therapy models are problem-focused, aiming to reduce dysfunction. While important, MRT aims to create conditions advocating for a sex-positive and pleasure-based approach. It distinguishes that sexual health and wellness are tied to the presence of pleasure, satisfaction, and the genuine expression of self. This aligns with the growing call in the sexual health field to move beyond a deficit model and embrace a broader vision of sexual wellness (Turner, 2020; Ford et al., 2019; Martos, 2016).

**Flexible Yet Structured**: MRT offers a clear, structured framework with its five tenets, providing a roadmap for assessment and intervention. It also allows for a great degree of flexibility. A therapist can fluidly move between addressing societal expectations, aligning values, analyzing and sharing power, and facilitating liberation, adapting to the client system's developmental needs. This flexibility is essential, as real-world therapy rarely follows a rigid, linear path.

**Promotes Fourth-Order Change**: MRT aims for "fourth-order change"—a fundamental redefinition of roles and relationships that extends beyond the therapy room into the community. It allows clients to change their behaviors and/or internal dynamics and transform their relational system while also empowering clients to practice and enact their new rules and dynamics from a place and stance of power.

**Advocacy and Legitimation**: In a world where Queer, Black, and Brown communities continue to face dehumanization and erasure, the recognition and utilization of MRT by therapists is an act of advocacy and legitimation. It creates a means not just for validation of these communities but for advancing the field forward to be more inclusive of diverse communities.

## An Inclusive Modality Toward Sexual Health

The progression of psychotherapy has revealed that humans value interconnectedness and that the space between us (i.e., our relationships) shape us. Sexual health is not an isolated domain sectioned off from other contextual factors. It touches multiple areas such as our individual psychology, our relational dynamics, our family histories, and the societal contexts in which we reside. MRT stands as an example of progress in this evolving landscape, offering a systemic model that is both theoretically rich and flexible.

By providing a clear and robust framework that explicitly addresses Societal Expectations, Values, Power Analysis, Liberation, and Radical Emancipation, MRT prepares sex therapists with the tools to navigate the complex challenges their clients face, particularly those from marginalized communities whose lived experiences are not readily found in therapeutic models.

As therapists, our commitment is to provide the most effective, attuned, and compassionate care possible. MRT, with its systemic foundation, integrative spirit, and unwavering commitment to justice, offers a powerful route to achieving this. By including MRT in your practice, we not only expand our clinical skills but also contribute to a more inclusive, equitable, and sexually affirming environments for all our clients.

**Exercises and Discussion Questions**

1 Examine your own knowledge regarding human sexuality and sex therapy training—what heteronormative assumptions might be embedded in techniques like sensate focus or communication exercises? How would you redesign these interventions from a queer-centered perspective?
2 This chapter describes moving from "tolerable sex" to vibrant sexual relationships through Radical Emancipation. How do you help clients envision and create sexual experiences that may have no precedent in their background or community? What does sexual "fourth-order change" look like practically?
3 MRT's approach to "societal expectations" in sex therapy involves challenging scripts about "normal" sexual behavior. How do you help clients distinguish between genuinely harmful sexual expectations and preferences that might seem unconventional but are healthy for them? Where do you draw ethical lines?
4 The integration of liberation and sex therapy means addressing how "internalized homophobia, transphobia, racism, and sexism" shape sexual experiences. How do you assess for these forms of internalized oppression in sex therapy? What specific interventions help clients reclaim sexual agency from oppressive narratives?
5 This chapter argues that MRT promotes "sex-positive and pleasure-based" approaches beyond dysfunction models. How do you shift therapeutic conversations from problem-focused to pleasure-focused while still addressing legitimate concerns? What training or personal work might therapists need to facilitate these conversations authentically?

# 14 The Future We're Building

## MRT in Community

### The Seeds Are Planted

Every revolutionary movement begins with a refusal. The refusal to accept that what is present must always be present. MRT began with my refusal to watch another Black Queer couple not have a model of therapy available that was reflective of their lived experiences or dynamics of wellness.

What started in my small therapy office with couples recapping their disdain in having to explain their lives and their experiences to previous therapists has grown into something I could not have imagined. Not because MRT has been presently validated by research or endorsed by institutions (those may come, or they may not), but because it speaks a truth that marginalized communities deserve to see within a field that is tasked with providing emotional and relational healing. Who you love does not need fixing. The systems that deny your humanity do.

The Colibri Center for Systemic Training (www.colibricentertraining.com) now serves as MRT's home base, but more importantly, it stands as a testament to what becomes possible when we center voices of color in psychotherapy. The center's mission extends beyond MRT, fundamentally reimagining therapy training and practice by asking: What if the voices pushed to the margins were brought to the center? What if accessibility wasn't an afterthought but the foundation? What if therapy training prepared clinicians not just to treat symptoms but to dismantle oppression?

Many therapists who have encountered MRT and its principles have shared in one form or another that a model like this helps them be more prepared to serve the Queer population. Many Black Queer couples and throuples who reads these principles and finally feel seen in a model of therapy. Every training program that finds a way to include this in their classes has become brave enough to challenge a Eurocentric curriculum. Many supervisors have stopped asking their supervisees to be "neutral" about oppression. Every community organization that adapts these principles for their healing circles; they all become invested in equity for all patrons, cultivating a future where therapy liberates rather than domesticates.

DOI: 10.4324/9781032725987-14

The seeds planted are not measurable by traditional research metrics. They're measured in the tears of recognition when a couple realizes they've been fighting each other instead of fighting oppression together. They're counted in the number of therapists of color who finally have language for why conventional models watered down their experienced truths.

## A Personal Reflection

As I write this conclusion, I sit with the weight and wonder of what MRT might become. I think about the couples who've shaped this model by bringing forward their courage in refusing to shrink, their creativity in building love from scratch, and their generosity in sharing their stories.

I think about Jamal and Marcus, who entered my office exhausted from code-switching and left as revolutionaries of love, now expecting their first child who will grow up with parents who refuse to hide. I think about Montana and Lamar, navigating interracial love and loss, who discovered that their differences were not problems to solve but strengths to celebrate. I think about the countless couples whose names I've changed for confidentiality but whose transformation changed me.

I think too about my own journey. How being a Black Queer first-generation American therapist is not just part of me but precious puzzle pieces of my life that have created a unique and beautiful collage. How every moment of marginalization became preparation for creating something new? How MRT is more than just my professional contribution but my love letter to every Black Queer person who was told their love was not real, was not valid, and was not worthy of celebration.

This model carries my hopes and the hopes of communities who have never had therapeutic models that centered the radiance that allowed them to shine. It carries the dreams of therapists of color who've been contorting themselves to fit into white frameworks. It carries the prayers of ancestors who loved boldly despite every attack against their lives.

MRT is personal because Radical Emancipation always is.

## The Future We Can Build Together

I envision a future that may not happen within my lifetime, but someday we see where:

## Therapy Transforms

- Every Black Queer couple can find a therapist will not retroactively fit their dynamics into models that do not fit their lived experiences and will celebrate their love.

- Therapy training programs require courses throughout the curriculum that ensure ample training in self of the therapist and cultural attunement.
- Payers such as insurance companies and governments recognize and cover culturally specific therapeutic approaches without requiring them to prove how they are "evidence-based" by white standards.
- Communities have emancipation centers and not just mental health clinics. These would be places where healing and revolution are synonymous.

## Practice Advances

- Therapists understand that neutrality in the face of oppression is complicity.
- "Cultural competence" is replaced by cultural attunement and structural analysis of power.
- Supervision includes examining how we perpetuate oppression, not just how we treat symptoms.

## Communities Heal

- Children grow up seeing all love as sacred.
- Families of origin learn to celebrate their Queer children rather than merely tolerate them.
- Black Queer love stories become templates for freedom, not cautionary or tragic tales.
- Radical Emancipation becomes as common as cognitive restructuring, thought stopping, and distress tolerance.

## Systems Shift

- Mental health organizations prioritize supporting and developing therapists from marginalized communities.
- Research centers study joy, resistance, and radical love as primary outcomes through qualitative means and is equal to the implementation of quantitative methodologies.
- Academic institutions recognize that the most innovative theories come from the margins.

This future requires collective dreaming and collective action. It requires therapists brave enough to abandon comfort, institutions willing to redistribute power, and communities bold enough to demand transformation rather than accommodation.

## The Invitation and the Challenge

This book concludes with both invitation and challenge, because revolution requires both welcome and disruption.

### *For Therapists*

**The invitation:** Join us in practicing therapy that liberates and bring the entirety of yourself. Your wounds, your wisdom, your identity into your work. Stop pretending that therapy can be apolitical when our clients' lives are politicized. Find your people at the Colibri Center, where voices of color lead and liberation is the curriculum.
**The challenge:** Examine how your practice might perpetuate oppression even with the best intentions. Question why you learned to privilege certain theories over others. Ask yourself who benefits from your "neutrality." Risk being "unprofessional" if professionalism means maintaining oppression.

### *For Training Programs*

**The invitation:** Integrate MRT and other models of therapy that are reflective of people of color into your curriculum. Hire faculty who embody these principles, not just study them. Create practicums and internship in communities that need revolution, not just treatment. Collaborate with the Colibri Center if there is a need to create curriculum that reflects this invitation.
**The challenge**: Realize that your curriculum may be producing therapists equipped to maintain the status quo rather than transform it. Acknowledge that "evidence-based" often means restrictive research methodologies and monolithic samples produce one-dimensional outcomes. Recognize that the communities most in need of healing are least represented in your theories, research, and faculty.

### *For Couples and Families*

**The invitation:** Know that a therapeutic model exists that centers your full humanity. Demand therapists who understand that your relationship challenges are both personal and political. Trust that your love whether it be whoever, however, and whenever is revolutionary. Share your liberation stories because others need to know freedom is possible.
**The challenge:** Release the internalized oppression that makes you believe you need fixing and that you are broken. Refuse therapy that asks you to adjust to systems designed for your destruction. Stop accepting therapeutic approaches that do not see your whole selves or the connected communities that promote growth and wellness. Expect more. Demand more.

### *For Researchers*

**The invitation:** Study what matters to marginalized communities. Develop assessment tools that capture liberation, joy, and other emotional and connected states that exist within Queer and communities of color. While the study of symptom reduction is helpful, we miss out on the qualitative expressions of connectedness that are protective factors. Include community impact in your effectiveness research. Center marginalized voices in research design, not just as subjects but as co-investigators in models such as Participatory Action Research.

**The challenge:** Question why certain outcomes are privileged over others. Ask who decided what counts as "evidence." Examine how research perpetuates oppression by studying marginalized people as problems rather than studying the systems that marginalize them. Help identify areas where systemic oppression exists and the positive impacts of revolution within communities.

## The Call to Action

The mental health field stands at a crossroads. We can continue practicing therapy that asks marginalized people to adjust to oppressive systems, or we can practice therapy that transforms those systems. We can maintain professional "neutrality" that sides with oppression, or we can take the radical stance that Liberation and Radical Emancipation are therapeutic avenues that need to be incorporated into every session treatment plan.

MRT will choose liberation every time.

This isn't easy work. You'll face resistance by choosing to practice from a model such as this. Resistance from colleagues who prefer comfort, from institutions protecting power, from insurance companies demanding pathology, sometimes from clients who've internalized oppression so deeply that freedom feels dangerous.

But you will not face it alone. The Colibri Center for Systemic Training (https://www.colibricentertraining.com/) offers more than MRT training. It provides:

- A community of revolutionary practitioners expanding the practice of systemic psychotherapy
- Training programs that center voices of color and lived experience
- Accessible spaces for therapists who've been marginalized by traditional institutions
- Person of the therapist (POTT) training and consultation groups
- Consultation groups where liberation is the lens
- Resources that prioritize community wisdom over academic jargon
- A vision of therapy that heals both individual wounds and collective trauma

More importantly, you'll be part of a lineage that has put in work to create pathways of liberty. You are joining ancestors who chose freedom despite consequence, elders who created Ballroom houses, Black Panthers who created programs to feed children and contemporaries building new worlds in therapy rooms and communities.

## Closing Meditation

Take a moment. Breathe. Feel the power within you.

Think about the couples you serve or will serve. Think about their struggles against systems that were never designed for their flourishing. Think about their resilience, their creativity, and their love persisting despite everything. Think about what becomes possible when therapy stops asking them to shrink and starts supporting them to soar.

Feel into your own body. Where do you hold the tension of oppression? Where do you carry the emotional exhaustion of code-switching? Where do you store the grief of unseen identity? Where do you hide the joy that feels too dangerous to show?

Now imagine. A therapy room where all of that is welcome. A therapeutic relationship where your liberation supports theirs. A model that says your existence is the qualification, not the liability. A future where therapy creates freedom, not adjustment.

That possibility and that permission is MRT's promise.

## A Final Offering

MRT is not complete, not perfect, and not for everyone. However, for those who have been waiting for a model that sees them, that centers them, and that believes in their capacity not just to heal but to transform, this is for you.

Take what serves you. Adapt what needs adapting. Challenge what needs challenging. Make it yours. Make it better. Make it work for the communities that you serve.

Because ultimately, MRT is more than following a manual or maintaining fidelity to a model. It's about a fundamental belief that the people most harmed by systems are the experts in transforming those systems. That love persisting despite oppression is the most powerful force for change. That therapy can be a liberation practice if practitioners become brave enough to make it so.

The revolution doesn't need permission. It doesn't need validation from institutions that were never designed to support it. It doesn't need evidence-based approval from systems invested in maintaining oppression. It just needs you. It needs your courage to practice differently. It needs your creativity to adapt and expand. It needs your commitment to liberation over comfort.

Welcome to the movement. We have been waiting for you. And together, we can move the field forward to be more inclusive.

# References


Absolon, K. (2010). Indigenous wholistic theory: A knowledge set for practice. *First Peoples Child & Family Review, 5*(2), 74–87.

Aponte, H. J. (2016). Supervision in the POTT Model. In H. J. Aponte & K. Kissil (Eds.), *The person of the therapist training model* (pp. 109–119). Routledge.

Aponte, H. J., & Kissil, K. (2014). "If I can grapple with this I can truly be of use in the therapy room": Using the therapist's own emotional struggles to facilitate effective therapy. *Journal of Marital and Family Therapy, 40*(2), 152–164. doi:10.1111/jmft.12011

Aponte, H. J., & Kissil, K. (Eds.). (2016). *The person of the therapist training model: Mastering the use of self.* Routledge.

Arlow, J. A. (1995). The "blank screen" and the analyst's subjectivity. *The Psychoanalytic Quarterly, 64*(2), 241–265. doi:10.1080/21674086.1995.11926615

Baird, S. (2021). *EMDR therapy and sexual health: A clinician's guide.* Springer Publishing Company.

Bausum, A. (2016). *Stonewall: Breaking out in the fight for gay rights.* Penguin.

Berry, M. D. (2013). The history and evolution of sex therapy and its relationship to psychoanalysis. *International Journal of Applied Psychoanalytic Studies, 10*(1), 53–74.

Betchen, S. J. (2013). *Intrusive partners-elusive mates: The pursuer-distancer dynamic in couples.* Routledge.

Black, L., & Jackson, V. (2005). Families of African origin. In M. McGoldrick, J. Giordano, & N. Garcia-Preto (Eds.), *Ethnicity and family therapy* (3rd ed., pp. 77–86). Guilford Press.

Branch, T. (1988). *Parting the waters: America in the king years* 1954–63. Simon and Schuster.

Brempong, A. (2000). The role of Nana Yaa Asantewaa in the 1900 Asante war of resistance. *Ghana Studies, 3*(1), 97–110.

Carmichael, S. (1966). Toward black liberation. *The Massachusetts Review, 7*(4), 639–651.

Carter, R. T., & Barket-San, J. S. (2015). Race-based and historical trauma: Implications for African American mental health. In A. T. H. Leong (Ed.), *Psychological trauma and the developing brain: An update on PTSD and its treatment* (pp. 43–58). Nova Science Publishers.

Carter, R. T., Johnson, V. E., Roberson, K., Mazzula, S. L., Kirkinis, K., & Sant-Barket, S. (2017). Race-based traumatic stress, racial identity statuses, and psychological functioning: An exploratory investigation. *Professional Psychology: Research and Practice, 48*(1), 30.

Campbell, M. E., & Herman, M. R. (2015). Both personal and public: Measuring interethnic marriage attitudes. *Journal of Social Issues, 71*(4), 712–732.

Chapman, G. (2009). *The five love languages: How to express heartfelt commitment to your mate*. Moody Publishers.

Collins, P. H. (1990). Black feminist thought in the matrix of domination. *Black Feminist Thought: Knowledge, Consciousness, and the Politics of Empowerment, 138*(1990), 221–238.

Comas-Díaz, L. (2016). Racial trauma recovery: A culturally sensitive treatment for posttraumatic stress disorder. *Journal of Multicultural Counseling and Development, 44*(1), 1–14. doi:10.1002/jmcd.12030

Comas-Díaz, L. (2020). Liberation psychotherapy. In L. Comas-Díaz & E. Torres Rivera (Eds.), *Liberation psychology: Theory, method, practice, and social justice* (pp. 169–185). American Psychological Association.

Crenshaw, K. (2019). 'Difference'through intersectionality 1. In *Dalit feminist theory* (pp. 139–149). Routledge, Taylor and Francis.

Davey, M. P., Davey, A., Tubbs, C., Savla, J., & Anderson, S. (2012). Second order change and evidence-based practice. *Journal of Family Therapy, 34*(1), 72–90.

Davis, A. Y. (1971). Political prisoners, prisons, and black liberation. *In If They Come in the Morning: Voices of Resistance* (pp. 27–43). Signet / New American Library.

DeGruy, J. (2005). *Post traumatic slave syndrome: America's legacy of enduring injury and healing*. Uptone Press.

Douglas, F. (2011). The traumas and tragedies of slave children and youth. In W. King (Ed.), *Stolen childhood: Slave youth in nineteenth-century America* (p. 212). Indiana University Press.

Du Bois, W. E. B. (2022). *The souls of Black folks*. Toronto Metropolitan University.

Duppong Hurley, K., Lambert, M. C., Gross, T. J., Thompson, R. W., & Farmer, E. M. (2017). The role of therapeutic alliance and fidelity in predicting youth outcomes during therapeutic residential care. *Journal of Emotional and Behavioral Disorders, 25*(1), 37–45.

Edwards, W. J. (2016). Measuring relationship satisfaction: Is it possible for black gay male couples to be satisfied in a relationship? *Deviant Behavior, 37*(8), 931–951. do i:10.1080/01639625.2016.1156983

Eldridge, K. A., & Christensen, A. (2002). Demand-withdraw communication during couple conflict: A review and analysis. In P. Noller & J. A. Feeney (Eds.), *Understanding marriage: Developments in the study of couple interaction* (pp. 289–322). Cambridge University Press.

Elliott, R., Bohart, A. C., Watson, J. C., & Murphy, D. (2018). Therapist empathy and client outcome: An updated meta-analysis. *Psychotherapy, 55*(4), 399.

Ellis, M. L., Weiss, B., Han, S., & Gallop, R. (2010). The influence of parental factors on therapist adherence in multi-systemic therapy. *Journal of Abnormal Child Psychology, 38*(6), 857–868.

Epstein, N. B., & Falconier, M. K. (2017). Shame in couple relationships. In J. Fitzgerald (Ed.), *Foundations for couples' therapy: Research for the real world* (pp. 374–383). Routledge, Taylor & Francis Group.

Everaerd, W., & Dekker, J. (1981). A comparison of sex therapy and communication therapy: Couples complaining of orgasmic dysfunction. *Journal of Sex & Marital Therapy, 7*(4), 278–289.

Fanney, R. (2005). *The last winter*. Dark Forest Press.

Flores, A. (2019). *Social acceptance of LGBT people in 174 countries, 1981 to 2017*. The Williams Institute.

Fonagy, P., & Luyten, P. (2019). Fidelity vs. flexibility in the implementation of psychotherapies: Time to move on. *World Psychiatry, 18*(3), 270.

Ford, J. V., Corona Vargas, E., Finotelli Jr, I., Fortenberry, J. D., Kismödi, E., Philpott, A., ... & Coleman, E. (2019). Why pleasure matters: Its global relevance for sexual health, sexual rights and wellbeing. *International Journal of Sexual Health, 31*(3), 217–230.

Gottman, J. M., & Gottman, J. S. (2013). Difficulties with clients in Gottman method couples therapy. In A. W. Wolf, M. R. Goldfried, & J. C. Muran (Eds.), *Transforming negative reactions to clients: From frustration to compassion* (pp. 91–112). American Psychological Association.

Hall, J. D. (2005). The long civil rights movement and the political uses of the past. *The Journal of American History, 91*(4), 1233–1263. doi:10.2307/3660172

Healy, R. W., & Allen, L. R. (2020). Bowen family systems therapy with transgender minors: A case study. *Clinical Social Work Journal, 48*(4), 402–411.

Hertlein, K. M., Weeks, G. R., & Gambescia, N. (Eds.). (2009). *Systemic sex therapy*. Routledge.

Hass-Cohen, N., Natrajan-Tyagi, R. R., & Arzt, J. (2017). Metacommunication in couple and family therapy. In J. Lebow, A. Chambers, & D. Breunlin (Eds.), *Encyclopedia of couple and family therapy* (pp. 1–6). Springer.

Hope, E. C., Brinkman, M., Hoggard, L. S., Stokes, M. N., Hatton, V., Volpe, V. V., & Elliot, E. (2021). Black adolescents' anticipatory stress responses to multilevel racism: The role of racial identity. *American Journal of Orthopsychiatry, 91*(4), 487.

hooks, B. (2006). *Outlaw culture: Resisting representations*. Routledge.

Jeffries, J. L. (2018). *On the ground: The Black Panther Party in a new era of black radicalism*. New York University Press.

Johnson, S. M., & Zuccarini, D. (2011). EFT for sexual issues: An integrated model of couple and sex therapy. In J. L. Furrow, S. M. Johnson, & B. A. Bradley (Eds.), *The emotionally focused casebook: New directions in treating couples* (pp. 219–246). Routledge, Taylor & Francis Group.

Jones, H. L., Cross Jr, W. E., & DeFour, D. C. (2007). Race-related stress, racial identity attitudes, and mental health among Black women. *Journal of Black Psychology, 33*(2), 208–231.

Jones, S. C., & Neblett, E. W. (2017). Future directions in research on racism-related stress and racial-ethnic protective factors for Black youth. *Journal of Clinical Child & Adolescent Psychology, 46*(5), 754–766.

Joseph, C. G. (2021). William Dorsey Swann. In H. L. Gates Jr. & E. B. Higginbotham (Eds.), African American national biography. Oxford University Press.

Joseph, P. E. (2006). *Waiting 'til the midnight our: A narrative history of black power in America*. Henry Holt and Co.

Kaplan, H. S., & Klein, D. F. (2014). Treatment: An integrated approach. In *Sexual aversion, sexual phobias and panic disorder* (pp. 84–124). Routledge, Taylor and Francis group.

Kaufman, J., Khan, M., Shepard Payne, J., Mancini, J., & Summers White, Y. (2023). Transgenerational inheritance and systemic racism in America. *Psychiatric Research and Clinical Practice, 5*(2), 60–73.

Kelledy, L., & Lyons, B. (2019). Circular causality in family systems theory. In J. L. Lebow, A. L. Chambers, & D. C. Breunlin (Eds.), *Encyclopedia of couple and family therapy* (pp. 431–434). Springer International Publishing.

Kidd, S. A., & Kral, M. J. (2005). Practicing participatory action research. *Journal of Counseling Psychology, 52*(2), 187.

Koffka, K. (2013). *Principles of Gestalt psychology*. Routledge.

Lebow, J., & Snyder, D. K. (2022). Couple therapy in the 2020s: Current status and emerging developments. *Family Process*, *61*(4), 1359–1385.

Lorde, A. (1984). *Sister outsider: Essays and speeches*. Crossing Press.

Lynn, M., Iftekhar, N., Adams, W., & Mumby, P. (2023). Multidisciplinary approach to the treatment of sexual dysfunction in couples using a biopsychosocial model. *The Journal of Sexual Medicine*, *20*(7), 991–997.

Martos, A. J. (2016). Vernacular knowledge and critical pedagogy: conceptualising sexual health education for young men who have sex with men. *Sex Education*, *16*(2), 184–198.

Masters, W. H., & Johnson, V. E. (1966). *Human sexual response*. Little, Brown & Company.

Masters, W. H., & Johnson, V. E. (1970). *Human sexual inadequacy* (Vol. 467, p. 58). Little Brown.

McCarthy, B., & Wald, L. M. (2017). A psychobiosocial approach to sex therapy. In Z. D. Peterson (Ed.), *The Wiley handbook of sex therapy* (pp. 190–201). John Wiley & Sons.

McDowell, T., Knudson-Martin, C., & Bermudez, J. M. (2019). Third-order thinking in family therapy: Addressing social justice across family therapy practice. *Family Process*, *58*(1), 9–22.

Merriam-Webster. (n.d.). Emancipation. In *Merriam-Webster.com dictionary*. Retrieved July 29, 2025, from https://www.merriam-webster.com/dictionary/emancipation

Mills, C. W. (2015). Bestial inferiority: Locating simianization within racism. *Simianization: Apes, Gender, Class, and Race*, *6*, 19.

Mize, S. J. (2015). A review of mindfulness-based sex therapy interventions for sexual desire and arousal difficulties: From research to practice. *Current Sexual Health Reports*, *7*(2), 89–97.

Mkabela, N. Q. (2015). The African philosophy of Ubuntu and its implications for indigenous psychology. *Journal of Psychology in Africa*, *25*(2), 127–133. doi:10.1080/14330237.2015.1027150

Muruthi, B., McCoy, M., Chou, J., & Farnham, A. (2018). Sexual scripts and narrative therapy with older couples. *The American Journal of Family Therapy*, *46*(1), 81–95.

Newton, H. P. (1973). *Revolutionary suicide*. Harcourt Brace Jovanovich.

Ngandu-Kalenga Greensword, S. (2022). Historicizing black hair politics: A framework for contextualizing race politics. *Sociology Compass*, *16*(8), e13015.

Nimbi, F. M., Galizia, R., Rossi, R., Limoncin, E., Ciocca, G., Fontanesi, L., ... & Tambelli, R. (2022). The biopsychosocial model and the sex-positive approach: an integrative perspective for sexology and general health care. *Sexuality Research and Social Policy*, *19*(3), 894–908.

Norcross, J. C., & Alexander, E. F. (2005). A primer on psychotherapy integration. *Handbook of Psychotherapy Integration*, *2*, 3–23.

Pantoja, S. (2020). Njinga a Mbande: Power and war in 17th-century Angola. In *Oxford research encyclopedia of African history*. Retrieved November 25, 2025, from https://oxfordre.com/africanhistory/view/10.1093/acrefore/9780190277734.001.0001/acrefore-9780190277734-e-326

Piot, P. (2006). AIDS: From crisis management to sustained strategic response. *The Lancet*, *368*(9534), 526–530.

Prasko, J., Ociskova, M., Vanek, J., Burkauskas, J., Slepecky, M., Bite, I., & Juskiene, A. (2022). Managing transference and countertransference in cognitive behavioral supervision: Theoretical framework and clinical application. *Psychology Research and Behavior Management*, *15*, 2129–2155. doi:10.2147/PRBM.S369294

Ransby, B. (2003). *Ella baker and the black freedom movement: A radical democratic vision*. University of North Carolina Press.

Schnarch, D. M. (1991). *Constructing the sexual crucible: An integration of sexual and marital therapy* (Vol. 550). WW Norton & Company.

Shepler, J. C., Glaros, A. G., & Boot, J. L. (2021). Minority stress and relationship satisfaction among gay and bisexual men. *Psi Chi Journal of Psychological Research, 26*(3), 296–306.

Skyttner, L. (1996). General systems theory: Origin and hallmarks. *Kybernetes*, *25*(6), 16–22.

Spengler, P. M., Lee, N. A., Wiebe, S. A., & Wittenborn, A. K. (2024). A comprehensive meta-analysis on the efficacy of emotionally focused couple therapy. *Couple and Family Psychology: Research and Practice*, *13*(2), 81.

Stevenson, B. E. (2023). *What sorrows labour in my parent'Ss breast?: A history of the enslaved black fSamily*. Rowman & Littlefield.

Tahan, M., Saleem, T., Moshtagh, M., Fattahi, P., & Rahimi, R. (2020). Psychoeducational Group Therapy for sexual function and marital satisfaction in Iranian couples with sexual dysfunction disorder. *Heliyon*, *6*(7), e04586.

Tate, K. (1998). *Black faces in the mirror: African Americans and their views on the American political system*. Princeton University Press.

Tripodi, F., Reisman, Y., & Lowenstein, L. (2022). The biopsychosocial approach in sexual medicine disorders. In Y. Reisman, L. Lowenstein, & F. Tripodi (Eds.), *Textbook of rare sexual medicine conditions* (pp. 7–18). Springer International Publishing.

Turner, G. W. (2020). The circles of sexuality: Promoting a strengths-based model within social work that provides a holistic framework for client sexual well-being. In M. Mohr-Carney, & A. Mendenhall (Eds.), *Rooted in Strengths: Celebrating the strengths perspective in social work* (pp. 305–325). University of Kansas Libraries.

Van Deburg, W. L. (1997). *New day in Babylon: The black power movement and American culture, 1965–1975*. University of Chicago Press.

Vargas, M. (2009). Fashion statement or political statement: The use of fashion to express black pride during the civil rights and black power movements of the 1960's. *Undergraduate Review*, *5*(1), 95–99.

Watzlawick, P., Weakland, J. H., & Fisch, R. (2011). *Change: Principles of problem formation and problem resolution*. WW Norton & Company.

Weeks, G. R. (2005). The emergence of a new paradigm in sex therapy: Integration. *Sexual and Relationship Therapy*, *20*(1), 89–103.

Weeks, G. R., Gambescia, N., & Hertlein, K. M. (2019). The intersystem approach to sex therapy. In K. M. Hertlein, N. Gambescia, & G. R. Weeks (Eds.), *Systemic sex therapy* (pp. 1–12). Routledge.

Westmacott, R., & Edmondstone, C. (2020). Working with transgender and gender diverse clients in emotion focused therapy: Targeting minority stress. *Person-Centered & Experiential Psychotherapies*, 19(4), 331–349.

Weiner, L., & Avery-Clark, C. (2014). Sensate focus: Clarifying the Masters and Johnson's model. *Sexual and Relationship Therapy*, *29*(3), 307–319.

Wiltsey Stirman, S. A., Gutner, C., Crits-Christoph, P. et al. (2015). Relationships between clinician-level attributes and fidelity-consistent and fidelity-inconsistent modifications to an evidence-based psychotherapy. *Implementation Science, 10*, 115. doi:10.1186/s13012-015-0308-z

Zarbo, C., Tasca, G. A., Cattafi, F., & Compare, A. (2016). Integrative psychotherapy works. *Frontiers in Psychology*, *6*, 2021.

# Appendix A

## Value Worksheet

**Directions:** This intervention can be done both in session with the couple or as homework. If completing the session as the therapist, go through each of the proposed listed values below and inquire each individual's viewpoint and write them down. This will allow for a proper ability to evaluate where and how the couple is aligned or divergent.

If requesting the couple to complete this session, they should look at the value in the center and write out their own individual thoughts on said topic.

The couple would then bring this completed form back to the next session for the therapist.

| *Partner 1* | *Value* | *Partner 2* |
|---|---|---|
| 1. ____________ | Money | 1. ____________ |
| 2. ____________ | Communication | 2. ____________ |
| 3. ____________ | Cleaning | 3. ____________ |
| 4. ____________ | Sex | 4. ____________ |
| 5. ____________ | Intimacy | 5. ____________ |
| 6. ____________ | Disagreements | 6. ____________ |
| 7. ____________ | Dependency | 7. ____________ |
| 8. ____________ | Independence | 8. ____________ |
| 9. ____________ | Family | 9. ____________ |
| 10. ____________ | Friends | 10. ____________ |
| 11. ____________ | Time spent | 11. ____________ |
| 12. ____________ | Career | 12. ____________ |
| 13. ____________ | Travel | 13. ____________ |
| ____________ | ____________ | ____________ |
| ____________ | ____________ | ____________ |
| ____________ | ____________ | ____________ |

Blank lines are included as the proposed values may not cover all of the topics that may cause a couple to be misaligned.

Feel free to enter in whatever topic that is therapeutically relevant.

# Appendix B

## Values Worksheet (Throuple)—Directions

**Directions:** This intervention can be done both in session with the throuple or as homework. If completing the session as the therapist, go through each of the proposed listed values below and inquire each individual's viewpoint and write them down. This will allow for a proper ability to evaluate where and how the throuple is aligned or divergent.

If requesting the throuple to complete this session, they should look at the value in the center and write out their own individual thoughts on said topic. The throuple would then bring this completed form back to the next session for the therapist.

| *Value* | *Partner 1* | *Partner 2* | *Partner 3* |
|---|---|---|---|
| 1. Money | | | |
| 2. Communication | | | |
| 3. Cleaning | | | |
| 4. Sex | | | |
| 5. Intimacy | | | |
| 6. Disagreements | | | |
| 7. Dependency | | | |
| 8. Independence | | | |
| 9. Family | | | |
| 10. Friends | | | |
| 11. Time spent | | | |
| 12. Career | | | |
| 13. Travel | | | |
| | | | |
| | | | |
| | | | |

Blank lines are included as the proposed values may not cover all of the topics that may cause a throuple to be misaligned.

Feel free to enter in whatever topic that is therapeutically relevant.

# Appendix C

## Power Analysis Walkthrough

| *Step 1: Analysis of Power* | *Step 2: Balance of Power* | *Step 3: Sharing of Power* |
|---|---|---|
| **Task 1: Identify who holds power in the system**<br>Therapist should work collaboratively with the client system to identify who holds power. | **Task 1: Hold critique of domination**<br>Therapist and relational unit should engage in health conversation regarding the possible use of Power Over as opposed of Power With. | **Task 1: Community care**<br>Therapist supports the relational unit to focus on care within the community and identify specific supports that the community may need to thrive. |
| **Task 2: Understand the sources of power**<br>Therapist should locate where (education, money, gender, sexual roles, etc.) the sources of power exist and they manifest in the system. | **Task 2: Exercise collective agency**<br>The relational unit is empowered to renegotiate a new understanding of how power can flow as they have shifted to Power With one another. | **Task 2: Inclusivity**<br>Therapist supports the relational unit to consider including other individuals that may have a direct impact on their community care (i.e., parents and friends) and ensure equality between one another in how power flows and is shared. |
| **Task 3: Map out the power in the system**<br>Therapist should map out the relationships between the partners, sources of power and the charge of each source (Negative, Equal, or Positive). See Appendix D for example. | **Task 3: Responsibility and accountability**<br>The therapist supports any redefinitions of roles and rules that help individuals and relational units to be responsible with power and build in accountability systems to broach conversations. | **Task 3: Justice**<br>Therapists support the relational unit to focus on ensuring actions are just and when infractions happen, they are taught how to repair. |
| **Task 4: Analyze power dynamics**<br>Therapist should work collaboratively to ensure a coherent understanding of the power dynamics is clear. | | |

# Appendix D

## Power Mapping Worksheet

**Directions:** Below is the Power Mapping grid. Each partner is assigned a column (a third column is included in case the relational unit is a throuple), and each row has space to enter in potential areas/topics that are sources of power. For each source, enter a (+) if that empowers the individual, enter a (−) if that individual does not receive power from source and enter a (=) if all individuals receive both powers equally from that source.

| *Source* | *Partner 1* | *Partner 2* | *Partner 3* |
|---|---|---|---|
| Gender presentation | | | |
| Mental health | | | |
| Education | | | |
| Money/wealth | | | |
| Career/job | | | |
| Community | | | |
| Family of origin | | | |
| Sexuality | | | |
| Sexual position | | | |

# Index

For Product Safety Concerns and Information please contact our EU representative GPSR@taylorandfrancis.com
Taylor & Francis Verlag GmbH, Kaufingerstraße 24, 80331 München, Germany

www.ingramcontent.com/pod-product-compliance
Ingram Content Group UK Ltd.
Pitfield, Milton Keynes, MK11 3LW, UK
UKHW020509130126
466905UK00004B/30

* 9 7 8 1 0 3 2 7 2 5 9 2 5 *